A HANDBOOK FOR PSYCHIATRIC NURSES

BY

T. ROBERTS

S.T.D., S.R.N., R.M.N., R.M.P.A.

Senior Tutor in Charge of the Psychiatric Nursing Area of the East Birmingham Group School of Nursing; Senior Nursing Officer (Teaching), Hollymoor Hospital, Birmingham

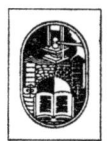

BRISTOL: JOHN WRIGHT & SONS LTD.

1971

Distribution by Sole Agents;
United States of America: The Williams & Wilkins Company, Baltimore
Canada: The Macmillan Company of Canada Ltd., Toronto

ISBN 0 7236 0303 0

PRINTED IN GREAT BRITAIN BY HENRY LING LTD., A SUBSIDIARY OF
JOHN WRIGHT & SONS LTD., AT THE DORSET PRESS, DORCHESTER

PREFACE

THIS handbook is, for convenience, divided into three sections: Section I, Human Development; Section II, Psychiatric; Section III, Medical. It is not in any way a textbook; it is merely a collection of useful information in note formation. Only the subject of Therapeutic Community in Section II has been elaborated upon beyond this point, and this is chiefly because it is somewhat an innovation in psychiatry.

It is thought likely that this book could be of special value to nurses working in psychiatric units of general hospitals, especially if they have not undertaken a recognized course of training in psychiatric nursing. Every attempt has been made to limit detail, and to concentrate instead on presenting an outline of the dominant features of a particular subject. Learning at the best of times is not an easy process, and this is not made any easier by the choice of textbooks available; many are too detailed. What the majority of psychiatric nurses favour is a handbook which can be read and understood easily and quickly, and which concentrates on basic essentials.

In Section I the emphasis is on emotional and social development and on highlighting the dominant behaviour pattern of various age-groups from birth to old age. Physical development has been omitted because of the relative unimportance of this to the work of the average psychiatric nurse.

In Section II an occasional diagram has been added here and there in an attempt to make certain abstract ideas more concrete. The dominant symptoms of the various mental illnesses are presented in the form of mnemonics, in the hope that those who like mnemonics as aids to memory will benefit from this. An attempt has been made to depart from the usual convention of starting with causes and following this with symptomatology etc. I consider that knowing about causes is of incidental importance to a nurse. Many textbooks for psychiatric nurses are written by psychiatrists, and this perhaps accounts for the convention. Psychiatrists do not always see things as the nurse does; I have therefore purposely added causes to the end of the section.

Section III covers in outline the more common forms of medical conditions which the psychiatric nurse may encounter. A study of medicine in depth requires, among other things, a thorough knowledge of human biology, chemistry, and pharmacology and can be very involved and time-consuming. Therefore, I believe that the best course for a nurse is to leave the technical detail to the expert, the specialist, and to concentrate instead on acquiring a working knowledge of the subject. There are plenty of reference books on the subject readily available in which to look up details and to check facts. Also there has been no attempt to elaborate beyond the basic clinical essentials. This, it is considered, is better learnt by precept at the bedside. Special reference is made to ward reporting and drugs only because they are the two subjects which seem to produce the most confusion and dispute at ward level. The value of this section lies not so much in the range of its content as in the choice and simplicity of the specific subjects which it contains.

The essential test of these notes will be in their practical use to the reader. They have already been of immeasurable value to me as a tutor and to many nurses with whom I have been associated over the last two decades. I sincerely hope that the reader will find this book helpful to an understanding and appreciation of psychiatry, psychology, psychiatric nursing, and basic clinical medicine. With use it could quite easily become a constant companion—a vade-mecum. It should also give much food for thought and serve to enhance the prestige and status of psychiatric nursing as a speciality *par excellence*.

Birmingham,   T. R.
June, 1971

CONTENTS

FOREWORD

By Elizabeth S. Bates, m.b., b.s., d.a.

*Clinical Assistant and Visiting Anaesthetist to a
Group of Psychiatric Hospitals*

With the modern trend of treating the mentally ill in psychiatric wards of general hospitals there has arisen a need for textbooks suitable not only for specialist psychiatric nurses but also for general nurses who are increasingly likely, either during training or later, to find themselves nursing psychiatric and psychogeriatric patients. A handbook of psychiatric nursing small enough to be readily portable but at the same time comprehensive enough to give instant help with everyday problems that occur is an invaluable adjunct to any nurse's personal library.

Although obviously useful to those undergoing psychiatric training and those returning to this specialty after an interval, this book will also be particularly helpful to those nurses undertaking a short form of psychiatric nursing as part of their general training. The sudden change from the structured discipline of the medical and surgical wards to what appears to be the more *laissez faire* atmosphere of the psychiatric unit is apt to leave the nurse temporarily at a loss as to her therapeutic role.

The short section on Human Development serves to promote an understanding of the psychiatric symptoms suffered by the mentally ill, while the descriptions of patient behaviour which results from these symptoms and the nursing techniques of use in the management of these patients, as set out in the Psychiatri-section, will aid the nurse not only in the psychiatric wards, but throughout her nursing career. Behaviour problems of psychoc logical origin are not confined to mental hospitals or psychiatric wards but are a frequent occurrence among the physically sick, as a study of the Medical section of this book will confirm.

Mr. Roberts has used a clear and simple style which should both teach and reassure all those with psychiatric nursing problems.

ACKNOWLEDGEMENTS

MATERIAL on psychosomatic illnesses has been extracted from Paul Kühne's *Medicine for the Layman* (trans. Jean Cunningham) by permission of Faber & Faber Ltd. Passages on neurosis and pre-clinical neurosis have been reproduced from *Mental Health and Environment* by Lord Taylor and Sidney Chave by permission of J. & A. Churchill Ltd.

SECTION I
HUMAN DEVELOPMENT

INTRODUCTION

IT is surprising how emotionally immature grown-ups become at times, although, from what I understand, only a small percentage of the general population is ever fully mature emotionally. The majority it seems is relatively immature. But as this is peculiar to the majority, it has to be accepted as normal and a feature of the average person.

Immaturity becomes abnormal only when it forms a social handicap. Naturally, there are degrees of immaturity relative to the age level at which emotional development has been arrested. When people act foolishly—and there are many adults who do this at times—they are advised either to grow up and be their age or to find something better to do; actually what is expected is that they become adults in the fullest sense. Unfortunately, however, all that can be hoped for in an adult who is childishly inclined is for some slight improvement in behaviour for a time.

Learning about the type of behaviour expected from childhood to old age is not only an absorbing study in itself, but also a useful yardstick for assessing behaviour and for comparing the behaviour of one person with that of another. Also to appreciate that not only may some of the patients that we look after be more intelligent than we are, but they may also be more emotionally mature, is an essential first step to accepting patients as people who merit our respect, protection, and understanding. Emotional maturity, however, bears very little relationship to intelligence, except in the sense that intelligence helps to modify behaviour and to check impetuosity.

A psychiatric nurse comes up against a good deal of immaturity in one form or another in the course of her work, and at times this can be most trying unless the nurse is mature enough herself to view this objectively and is able to accept it sensibly as a matter of course. It sometimes helps to get into the habit of describing a patient as being of low maturity rather than immature. To say that he is immature is apparently too absolute and dogmatic and is not, therefore, conducive to promoting tolerance and goodwill. Like all dogmatic assertions, it condemns more than it commends. Students of human behaviour especially may do well to bear this in mind.

3

DEVELOPMENT AND GROWTH

Development is a process of gradual growth involving an organized series of changes necessary for allowing a structure to fulfil an essential function. Development is genetically controlled, but strongly influenced by the environment.

Growth is the increase in size and weight of a structure and is controlled mainly by the endocrine glands.

Development starts from conception and continues for several years after birth. Development occurs on four main levels:—

    i. Physical.
    ii. Emotional.
    iii. Intellectual.
    iv. Social.

General characteristics of living things. What are they ? See if you can make a list of these for yourself. Also, what do living things need to keep alive and to remain healthy ?

CHILDHOOD

Characteristics of an Infant at Birth

A bundled mass of restless activity with strong hand grasping and sucking reflexes.

Dependent and helpless.

Needs protection from injury, infection, dehydration, malnutrition, and from neglect in general.

It also needs water, food, oxygen, comfort, shelter, warmth, rest, affection, and the security of a regular pleasant and comforting routine.

It makes known its many needs through crying and distress.

At about 3 weeks after birth, the average child begins to differentiate between itself and the environment, and to identify 'me' and the 'not me'.

At about the age of 3 months, when it becomes able to fix its eyes on objects and to respond to sounds, it acquires greater awareness of its environment.

Characteristics of an Infant up to the Age of 6 Months

Dependent.
Needs mothering continuously.
Easily distressed.

Begins to respond constructively to the environment through reaching out for things.

Behaviour, however, is instinctual and follows a cyclical pattern, e.g., sleeping, incontinence, waking up, crying, hunger, feeding, comforting, sleeping.

It makes use of simple substitutes such as thumb-sucking when hungry or in need of comfort.

Every living person has, apart from physical needs such as a need for water, food, oxygen, etc., a number of basic psychological needs. These, which include security, affection, recognition, and responsibility, have to be satisfied if healthy development is to be established and maintained.

The need for responsibility is, of course, unimportant in the first 12 months or so.

Characteristics of a Child from 6 Months to 2 Years

Instinctual desires are still dominant.

He lives somewhat mechanically through his special senses.

Interpretation of the environment is unrealistic and limited to his immediate surroundings.

He is highly self-centred, self-willed, and destructive.

Shows distress and aggression easily when frustrated.

He thinks in wholes, and is not capable of reasoning, mainly because he is only able to appreciate one thing at a time.

He is, however, quite able to turn a blind eye to what he may dislike.

This seems to be a built-in defence mechanism that automatically helps to protect him from distress.

He is, of course, highly impressionable and suggestible.

Learning is based mainly on trial and error.

Characteristics of a Child from 2 to 5 Years

As his intelligence is gradually developing, he becomes more able to learn and use new skills. He is also more able to use reason in his social adjustments. When his wants are restricted or frustrated he may become awkward and difficult. He may refuse food, have temper tantrums, wet himself, bite his nails, refuse to communicate, may withdraw, become passive and socially apathetic.

At this age he is more realistic in his awareness and approach to things in the world around him.

He is very curious and enjoys imitating his parents and loves to explore around the house.

Characteristics of a School-age Child

He is now a small version of his parents.
He is becoming more independent.
Has more self-discipline and self-assurance.
He is adventurous and puts on a bold front.
He is proud of himself and loves to show off.
He is curious to master the unfamiliar and the unknown.
While he is brave and bold in the light of day, he still turns to his mother during the hours of darkness.

Some Difficulties that a Child may experience

1. DURING THE FIRST 2 YEARS

These are concerned with feeding, teething, walking, habit training, sleeping.

2. BETWEEN 2 AND 5 YEARS

Difficulty in controlling his aggression and learning to give and take, especially with other children.

Having to come to terms with such feelings as anger and jealousy.

3. SCHOOL-AGE CHILD

Overcoming fear of other children or of going to school.

Feeling of inferiority.

Physical difficulties such as partial blindness, deafness, poor and weak physique, short stature, and deformity.

Social difficulties may arise from the attitude of other children and of other people, including teachers, to him.

Finding it difficult to learn to keep up with other children, and to satisfy the aspirations of parents.

Unfavourable features which may be detected in the behaviour of a child may include one or more of the following:—

Hyperactivity and restlessness.
Demanding and impatient attitude.
Aggressive reactions.
Temper tantrums.
Unwillingness to participate in play.
Fear of other children.
Doubt of self-value.
Tics, e.g., blinking and other mannerisms.

These are unfavourable in that they may interfere with normal social development and adjustments.

How to help a Difficult Child

1. Try to work out why the child is difficult.
2. Try to accept that it is probably your fault.
3. Do not laugh at a child, laugh with him.
4. Always give adequate knowledge to the child and do not avoid matters of sex. Try to forget your own taboos about sex.
5. Beware of always nagging and running the child down.
6. Never criticize a child in front of his friends.
7. Aim at trying to say, 'Well done, you cannot do better than your best'.
8. Allow the child to play with other children.
9. Beware of worrying about table manners.
10. Let the child grow up to rely upon himself.

The emotional insecurity of children may be expressed as either a disorder of habit, a disorder of conduct, or a disorder of personality.

Disorders of habit include nail-biting, thumb-sucking, stammering, incontinence, or refusal to pass faeces.

Disorders of conduct include wandering, temper tantrums, lying, stealing, truancy, refusing to eat.

Disorders of personality include day dreaming, undue sensitivity, obstinacy, stubbornness, sullenness, over-activity, inhibition, excitability, excessive fastidiousness, etc.

Features of a Healthy Child

He is active, energetic, curious, adventurous, and out to prove himself.

Adjusts easily to new situations.

Seeks friends and company and plays well and happily with other children.

Able to take the rough with the smooth in competitive play.

Has confidence and assertiveness.

Learns to create more than he destroys.

Loves to experiment and to find how things work.

Responds easily to kindness and affection.

The Deprived Child

This is usually a description of a child deprived of love, affection, and emotional security in the mother–child relationship.

(What do you consider is the difference between being affectionless and unaffectionate ?)

Children on the whole respond to loss or to withdrawal of love with hostility and distress, and many rebel most violently.

As time goes on, however, and if the deprivation persists, rebellion may quite easily give way to passivity and emotional aloofness. This is a defensive response and is an attempt to turn a blind eye to a painful experience. It is only by recreating or restoring a loving relationship with the child that one can ever hope to prevent total withdrawal. This is imperative and the sooner it is done the better, if injurious effect on the personality is to be avoided.

Relationship between Mother and Child

The normal relationship between mother and child should be pleasant and emotionally satisfying, even though it may at times be laborious, demanding, and time-consuming.

A healthy relationship establishes a climate of mutual acceptance and one which is conducive to fostering trust, security, happiness, and contentment. Both mental health and normal development of the child's personality depend upon it. Failure to satisfy basic needs at this time is therefore detrimental to future normal development. In an attempt to satisfy both physical and emotional needs of the child, the mother has to give a good deal of herself and usually this is what the average mother does unstintingly with pride, joy, and tenderness.

Discipline and the Child

Discipline is the control which the child is able to accept from parents, and which after a time he is able to apply himself without direction. At first, control is unavoidably authoritarian, because at this age the child is not able to reason things out fully for himself. But as he develops he soon appreciates why certain things are or are not permitted. At this stage, discipline is related to approval and disapproval and to the child's own level of appreciation. It is from this that the child applies self-discipline. The control which the child acquires over himself and his environment is reflected in the stability and predictability of his actions.

THE REQUISITES FOR HEALTHY DISCIPLINE
1. Good examples.
2. Sincerity, trust, consistency, and approval.

3. Respect for individuality.
4. Satisfaction of basic needs.
5. Routine and uniformity.

What do you consider are the values of discipline?

Emotional Development

In the healthy child, emotions seem to develop in a definite sequence, with distress as the first emotion to appear.

Excitement, disgust, anger, fear, delight, jealousy, and joy are others which appear in the first 2 years and this is the order in which they appear. Some are more susceptible to emotional stimulation than others, and this, it seems, is part of their make-up —their temperament.

The normal well-adjusted person should be able to respond to people and situations with pleasantness and confidence and without undue anxiety, indecisiveness, and aggressiveness.

The following are some of the emotional responses which may be seen in both children and adults alike:—

ANXIETY

Where there is a readiness to become unduly tense, keyed-up, and to make big things out of small things.

OBSESSIONAL

Where the person cannot make up his mind easily, and is usually over-conscientious and fussy over details.

AGGRESSIVE

Where the person is touchy, suspicious, and ready to take offence.

ROLE-TAKING

Where the person dramatizes situations unnecessarily. Seeks limelight and identifies himself completely with other people.

Social Development

This is supposed to occur in three stages:—

1. The stage of aloofness.
2. The stage of conflict and hostility.
3. The stage of co-operation.

The emotionally balanced child reaches the final stage easily and quickly. It is the insecure, deprived, and neglected child who may find this difficult. Quite a number become arrested at the second stage. Much patience, tact, and understanding, therefore, is required to overcome the resistance and hostility experienced at this stage.

PLAY

First and foremost, play is essential for normal social development. Through play a child is able to release aggression, to satisfy curiosity, and to use his imagination creatively. He is also able to experiment with and to manipulate things. He acquires skills and develops initiative. It gives pleasure to the senses and muscles, widens social contacts, provides companionship, and gives the child an understanding of his environment. Through play a child learns to distinguish between the real and the unreal and acquires muscle co-ordination, discipline, and self-confidence.

A child's play, it is considered, serves the same biological function as dreams; it helps to solve problems. This it does through repetitive activity and acting out.

The type of play follows the various stage of maturation. Between the ages of 1 and 4 years play takes the form of peep-bo and hide and seek. Between 4 and 7 years play becomes more dramatic and it is expressive of individuality, with one child playing the role of a queen, etc.

With the onset of the grouping stage, at 8 years or thereabout, play becomes more socially organized. Now the child directs its energies to camping, cycling, and swimming with friends. One thing about play is that on the whole it is not organized by rules. Once we introduce rules, we shift the emphasis from play to games.

IN-BETWEEN YEARS OF CHILDHOOD (6–12 YEARS)

Characteristics (Supplementary to Characteristics of the School-age Child, p. 6)

School plays an important part in their lives.

New grown-ups become exciting and interesting in their own right, instead of being like their parents.

The world of other children with its games, gossip, secrets, rivalry, and admirations becomes his world.

At first, experiences mixed feelings about mother—e.g., doubting if she is his real mother or not. This makes him unhappy and angry.

Bouts of agonizing homesickness may attack some children when they are first away from home. This may be especially prolonged in those who still feel guilty over their occasional angry feelings towards their parents.

Become dependent and wanting affection when they are tired or ill.

For the most part, when healthy they appear self-reliant, cocky, and superior, much more so than they really are.

They want to be active and doing all the time.

They are full of ideas and questions about what makes things tick in the world about them.

Not willing to talk about their secret feelings and fantasies.

They have their own way of dealing with problems.

All sorts of compulsive behaviour are common (having to walk over cracks between paving stones, having to touch certain objects, having to be out of the lavatory before the flush has finished running, etc.). These are all magic ways of dealing with anxiety.

Become very aware of the wrong-doing of others.

Turn a blind eye towards their own shortcomings.

They are 'tell-tales', but these tales shouldn't be taken too seriously.

Games of counting, of bodily skills, and competition are common, and counting out games still persist. (These are ways of finding out one's place in the world and of trying to impose order and control on impulses and feelings without having to think the matter out.)

Crazes come and go.

Pockets, drawers, and bedrooms are full of strange objects, which must not be thrown away or touched.

Clothes are dropped as they are taken off, because there is always some private concern which must be attended to immediately.

Tend to accept other people's standards instead of those of their parents.

If they cannot get their own way, they tend to say ' But the others are allowed to do it. Why shouldn't I ?'

Apparent indifference to parental standards is most upsetting.

This is an important stage in life in which they need help in building up ideas of desirable behaviour, help in establishing efficient defences against their unruly impulses and a conscious and reasonable self-control.

Values need to be discussed constantly, choice of behaviour given, but control and authority maintained, sometimes quite strictly.

THE GANG

Between the ages of 8 and 15 years, both boys and girls come together in loosely organized groups, on equal terms and at random. At puberty, however, the pattern changes; the group becomes now more selective and homosexual. This is the gang stage.

The formation of gangs is a natural impulse and is held together by a common interest such as football, or beating up rival gangs. A well-established gang, held together by a common loyalty to a leader, may exist for many years.

INTELLECTUAL DEVELOPMENT

Intelligence is an all-round mental efficiency which develops gradually up to the age of 15 to 20 years. It is characterized by the ability to see relationships between facts not particularly studied or considered before, and is also associated with creativeness and foresight.

It helps us to improve on our performance and to benefit from experience.

It helps us to adjust quickly to a new environment.

Enables us to detect absurdities.

It is through intelligence that we create a new situation and reorganize the old system and method.

Intelligence can be tested and is often expressed as the I.Q. (intelligence quotient). This is the ratio between the mental age of the individual and his chronological age. The result is multiplied by 100.

$$\frac{M.A.}{C.A.} \times \frac{100}{1}$$

The I.Q. ranges from one extreme to the other: 100 is taken as the average; mental subnormality below 75; very superior above 130.

After the age of 30 years, intelligence gradually declines, but this is not appreciably noticeable because of the wisdom and experience which influences our outlook.

It has been said that after the age of 20 years the brain begins to lose about 1 g. a year in weight and that about 30 brain-cells die every minute, probably never to be replaced.

Stages in the development of intelligence in children educated to use numbers, etc., are significant as follows:—

AGE 3
    Show me your nose.
    Repeat 2 numbers after me.
AGE 4
    Repeat 3 numbers.
    Count 4 pennies.
AGE 5
    Copy a square.
    Perform 3 commissions.
    Copy a diamond.
    Name 4 primary colours.
    Repeat 4 numbers.
AGE 6
    Count 13 pennies.
    Copy sentence 'See little Paul'.
    Define concrete terms—'What is a fork?'
    Name the days of the week.
AGE 7
    Writing from dictation.
    Count pennies and 3 halfpennies.
    Repeat 5 numbers.
AGE 8
    Count backwards from 20 to 0.
    Give the full date.
    Name the months.
AGE 9
    Repeat 6 numbers.
AGE 10
    Build a sentence with 3 words.
    Draw 2 designs from memory.
AGE 11
    Detect absurdities.
    Repeat 7 numbers.
AGE 12
    Rearrange mixed sentences—'a defends dog good his bravely master'.

PUBERTY AND ADOLESCENCE

Puberty is the stage of sexual awakening which precedes adolescence, whilst adolescence itself, as a stage of rapid growth and development, is a transitional phase which transforms a child into an adult. On average this lasts about 6 years from about the age of 12 years until or just beyond the age of 18 years, and may for convenience be divided into three periods—early, middle, and late adolescence.

Characteristics of Adolescence

PHYSICAL

Body changes are easily visible.

In girls, breasts become prominent, hips widen, and menstruation begins.

Boys seem to 'shoot up' rapidly and become taller than the average girl. The voice changes and semen is produced by the testes.

Hair and fat become distributed characteristically in each sex, and in one respect the distribution of hair is obvious in the smoother, hairless face of the girls.

MENTAL

Adolescence may be described as a rebellious, passion-laden, identity- and role-seeking phase. Hero worshipping is quite common.

Many doubt the wisdom of adults and tend to oppose and to reject the conventional standards. Instead they set up their own.

In outlook they are likely to be bombastic, critical, arrogant, self-opinionated, energetic, and full of self-display.

They have definite views about ways of living, about sex, religion, education, authority, clothes, and so on.

Clothes, though extreme in style and fashion, are generally colourful and gay.

Inwardly they feel insecure, inferior, ignorant, and self-conscious.

Many are often sensitive, moody, irritable, restless, and easily bored.

Some are highly conscious of their personal appearance and become preoccupied with style of hair, shape of nose, size of feet, and so on.

It is therefore of little surprise that so many girls attempt to hide their faces, not to mention their spots, with their hair.

Adolescents need reputation, company, something or someone to respect and to admire, sympathy, encouragement, opportunity to excel and to achieve something worthwhile.

They need to be emotionally independent and to be sexually active. They also need an outlet for their excess energy and for their adventurous spirit.

The Attitude of Many Adolescents to Work may be associated with:—

1. Making a lot of money quickly.

2. Deceiving the boss as much as possible.

3. Thinking that he who does the least work is the most successful.

4. Working only if the boss works.

5. As they experience jealousy easily, they find it difficult to praise other young people of their own age.

In their attempt to be independent, adolescents resent criticism and direct supervision. They much prefer to find things out for themselves. Many, however, respond well to suggestions, and though they may be highly self-centred they are quite capable of giving a good deal of themselves to a worth-while cause if managed wisely.

Some of the Problems that may be encountered by Adolescents

PERSONAL

1. A strong feeling of inferiority and inadequacy.

2. Feeling fatigued and lacking in stamina, concentration, and stickability.

3. Overpowering self-consciousness and self-absorption.

4. A feeling of loneliness with a strong sense of rejection.

5. Not knowing how best to remain loyal to the standards of parents while trying to create their own standards and personal identity.

6. Boredom through inactivity.

7. Being in constant need of reassurance.

8. Sexual maladjustment.

SOCIAL

1. Being misunderstood by adults.

2. Being constantly blamed for clumsiness and awkward behaviour.

3. Not being able to find sufficient outlet for superfluous energy.

4. Undue embarrassment and apprehension on meeting people.

5. Anti-authoritarian outlook with a constant desire to challenge time-honoured customs and established order.

6. Inadequate outlet with resulting misdirection of the spirit of adventure, eagerness to experiment, exhibitionism, and excitability.

7. Bombastic, rash, risky, daring, brash, impulsive behaviour with a self-opinionated attitude preventing normal adjustment to and acceptance of other people.

8. Inability to find stable employment.

9. Inability to get on with the opposite sex.

10. Ineducability, retarding progress.

11. Passionate love affairs.

12. Morbid preoccupation with physical features and appearance.

ADULTHOOD

The emergence of the adult from the restless world of adolescence is a gradual process, which the majority of young people manage quite easily.

An adult is expected to be well adjusted, alert, assertive, and independent, and capable of holding his own against the many ups and downs of life with persistence, stamina, and equanimity.

An adult, if emotionally matured, has a wide range of interests, displays spontaneous emotional control, and is able to make satisfactory adjustment to distress with ease. And, if mentally healthy as well, he is optimistic, sociable, and able to display emotions spontaneously and naturally, without swinging to the extreme.

Overall the average adult is happy, enjoys life, and is genuinely interested in the opposite sex and derives fulfilment from family life.

Courtship

This is an essential prologue to marriage. It is a trial and a testing period, and as they woo and possess each other with charm, sympathy, protective tenderness, patience, tolerance, and pleasantness, they come to find out if they are compatible or not.

In one respect courtship may be viewed as an exercise in self-display and in presenting the most attractive side of one's nature. Courtship should last from six to twelve months at least, to allow for attraction to qualities other than physical ones.

It is considered that a man wants company and affection from a woman whilst a woman wants generosity, kindness, and love from a man.

Happiness and contentment depend upon this. It is also essential for each to appreciate and respect those attributes and qualities which are determined by sex and which make the man different from the woman and vice versa, without competition.

Marriage

There are many reasons why people get married. It may be, apart from an instinctive need to mate, because:—

1. It is considered the right and proper thing to do.
2. The couple are really in love and are unable to do without each other any longer.
3. One or both partners need support and protection.
4. Of a possible economic advantage—marrying into money, for example.
5. Of a desire for revenge against a dictatorial parent.
6. Of insecurity and a fear of being 'left on the shelf'.
7. Of illegitimacy.
8. They desire to have children.
9. They have been pushed into it by their parents.

SUCCESS OF MARRIAGE

There is no special formula for this. Basically it is a matter of compromise and much depends upon the compatibility of temperaments.

However, there are a number of factors which have direct bearing on the success of marriage and these include:—

1. The relative intelligence of the married couple. If one has a good deal more intelligence than the other, it could create difficulty, unless there is a considerable amount of patience and give and take between the two.

2. The reason for getting married. Was it a 'shot-gun' wedding, or was it really based on true love?

3. The presence of or the prospects of having children. Children strengthen the bonds of marriage. They widen the field of interest within the family. They counteract selfishness and bring fresh interest into what might otherwise become a dull, self-centred, and selfish household. Children force an issue of responsibility on the partners. They also supply a definite purpose and a good reason for having to sacrifice and for working hard.

4. The personalities of the married couple. Immaturity often creates a fickle unstable relationship, particularly if the immature person is also possessive and self-centred. Opposite temperaments, however, often complement each other and seem to work out quite well. One example of opposites would be the quiet and the boisterous.

A family is a closed group with a pattern of behaviour peculiar to itself and to its members. No two families are ever alike, even though there may be similarities.

ADVANTAGES OF BELONGING TO A FAMILY GROUP

Because of the intimacy and identification which exists within the average family, members are able to relax and to forget many of the problems and cares of the world outside. Being a member of a happy family brings contentment and security.

A family also gives opportunity for learning skills and habits of generations past. These are usually handed down from parent to child, almost endlessly. This is therefore an essential means of propagating our culture and our way of life.

A well-integrated family is also protective and is able, through its planned economy, to make sure that no one member goes short of anything. It therefore serves to satisfy needs and wants of individuals.

And whilst some may accept family life as a bastion of a civilized community, others would oppose this on the grounds that, because of its stereotyped form, family life retards progress.

GROWING OLD

The body reaches its peak of efficiency before the age of 30 years. After this, efficiency declines. At first, apart from a few extra wrinkles, this is relatively imperceptible. It is only after the age of 40 years that we become aware of loss of efficiency and of the changes which are taking place in the body.

Ageing is a gradual process of deterioration, evident in greying hair, receding hair in men, wrinkled skin, reduced stamina, and the tendency to put on body fat. The decline in intelligence, however, is compensated for by increased wisdom and is noticeable only in the difficulty which older people have in learning and retaining new facts.

The period between 40 years and 50 years of age is a period of depression, anxiety, confusion, and conflict for many people. For, as they become aware of ageing and the aches which accompany this, they tend to become cynical and unduly preoccupied with future prospects and the thought of dying. General well-being, therefore, depends upon the ease with which they adjust to and resolve these many problems.

Women, as they approach the climacteric stage, may suffer from headaches, hot flushes, irritability, and loss of interest, as well as anxiety and depression, already referred to. These symptoms are due to the imbalance of hormones in the body. The lack of oestrogen (the hormone from the ovary) may be corrected by oral administration. Correcting this clears up many of the symptoms experienced at this time.

OLD AGE

Loss of weight is now more definite, and as the body dries up and the subcutaneous fat disappears, the skin becomes dry and wrinkled and the eyes sunken and lustreless. Bones become brittle whilst teeth decay and loosen. Movements become slow, awkward, and difficult, and with increased stubbornness and querrulousness, they begin to neglect their many responsibilities and become difficult to manage. As this is in general a period of social isolation, they feel, and are, very lonely.

The two things which they dread above all else are loneliness and poverty. And as their memory for recent events fails, they become progressively absent-minded and talk incessantly of days long past.

As senior citizens they need respect, security, and help to maintain their dignity and independence. And as they become house-bound and unable to care for themselves, they will need more than a few kind words—they will need real companionship and practical help with supervision.

SECTION II

PSYCHIATRIC

INTRODUCTION

HAVE you ever felt restless and jittery, and felt as if you were going off your rocker? If you have, take heart, for there are thousands of people like you. Some may be standing or sitting beside you right now. Take a look. Can you tell? I doubt it, for you need a good deal of experience and training for this, and even then you cannot always be certain of what you see. Imagination plays havoc with the best of us.

It is surprising how many people there are with worries, doubts, fears, and other similar problems. It is estimated that between 30 and 35 per cent of the population suffer at times from a combination of depression, attack of nerves, irritability, and sleeplessness. It is little wonder that there is a run on sleeping pills and tranquillizers. These must be swallowed by the thousand. People who experience these problems are usually unhappy people, even though they do not always let on that they are so. For as they fight to survive with all their might they manage reasonably well, even though this may be at the expense of their eating and sleeping, to put on a smile and to keep up appearances. Just think how much of themselves they must sacrifice to keep this up. It is indeed an endless struggle and a strain which only the strongest can bear without a nervous breakdown.

A few unfortunately do break under the strain, and these are the few who become some of the many whom we are able to help and to look after in a mental hospital. About 1 in 14 of the population will, in their lifetime, spend some time in hospital under psychiatric care.

It is amazing how ignorant many people are about what goes on in a psychiatric hospital. People have all sorts of weird ideas. They still cannot accept that a mental hospital is a hospital just like any other, except that because of the nature of the illness there are fewer patients being nursed in bed.

Our patients are up and about and are, with expert help, actively engaged in trying to sort out their emotional and social difficulties. The majority of patients in a mental hospital are not spectacular. They do not rave or scream or tear their hair. Their memories are good. They answer questions sensibly and they talk convincingly. Many are probably more intelligent than we are.

Mental hospitals today are no longer drab and dreary places; they are now bright and cheerful with standards of decor and comfort which may better what we ourselves have at home.

The main difficulty which many of our patients experience is in not being able to get on with other people, especially outside the hospital. Naturally, many are awkward through being either absent-minded, unduly suspicious, down in the dumps, a little over-excited, indifferent to the world around them, or excessively fearful of travelling on buses and so on.

But, when you think of it, these are not all that far removed from what you or I may experience at times. The difference is often only one of degree. However, we can always declare that because we are able to adjust socially more easily, we are more normal and therefore more socially acceptable than they are. But whether we have the right to claim this or not, is another matter.

It often seems that once a person has lost his usefulness to society, he is no longer *persona grata*, and that the only thing to do is to get rid of him. Push him out of the way. Incarcerate him if necessary. Do what you will, as long as you leave us—the 'hale and hearty'—alone, to pursue our life in peace and comfort. We will pity, yes, and we will give a few shillings towards this cause and that, but beyond this leave us alone. We have enough to do, looking after ourselves. What magnanimous sentiment!

This sort of selfish indifference has been with us for a very long time, and in days gone by especially, it was in part responsible for locking people up in what were then called asylums. Today, there are no asylums with padded rooms and bars across the windows. Instead we have hospitals in the fullest sense. Doors are open and patients are free to move in and out at will.

The critism now, of course, is that we are giving our patients too much freedom; whilst this may be justifiable in some cases, it is not on the whole a valid criticism. In my opinion it springs from the prejudices and intolerance towards mental illness which are still prevalent in the community. We still have not been able to convince the public that mental illness is an illness like any other, that a mental hospital is a hospital, that mental patients are sick people, not lunatics, and that mental nurses are nurses in their own right.

Psychiatric nursing is unique in that it offers opportunities not available in many other jobs. This is mainly because nurses do things for, to, and with people. Just imagine the personal satisfaction and pleasure this brings. Through their relationships with people psychiatric nurses get to know a great deal about people and their behaviour.

You must agree, we are all concerned with trying to find reasons and explanations for why people act in the way they do. This is an absorbing pursuit, and it is little wonder that so many of those who become psychiatric nurses find this and the care of the mentally sick so rewarding. Also, just think of the self-confidence one gains through active participation in group functions and social relationships of all forms.

From one angle a nurse's job in a psychiatric hospital is really quite simple. To be an efficient nurse, you need only to bear in mind that, though the patients are sick and we are well, at rock bottom they need the same things as we do: a decent place to live, comfort, personal cleanliness, suitable clothing, nourishing, well-served food, exercise, work and fun, and sleep. These add up to the normal life, the good life. Everyone needs to be physically and mentally well. But, in its details, the work is far from simple. Doing it well and easily takes the best of any man's or woman's brains, character, and imagination.

Consider the amount of skill and understanding you would need to restore confidence, personal pride, and a desire to get well, in a person who is totally indifferent to the world around him. You could even go as far as saying that socially he is 'dead'. There's a problem and a challenge for you. Also, if in every fat man there is a thin man trying to get out, might not there be a healthy man trying to get out of every unhealthy one. If this is so, then what we may have to do first is to wake the healthy beggar up and this, as you can well imagine, is not the easiest of tasks. Actually, what we attempt to do with many of our patients is to rouse their desire to get well. Sometimes, this is like trying to get blood out of stone.

This, you might say, is a job for the expert; and so it might well be, for in psychiatry we have at least three types of experts. There is the psychiatrist, who is the expert in mental illness and its treatment, then the psychologist, the expert who knows more than anyone else about the human mind, and thirdly the nurse, who by virtue of her training and experience is an expert in human relationships. All three work together as a team in an attempt to restore a healthy mind to a healthy body, and a healthy person to a healthy society.

MENTAL HEALTH

Mental health is so closely tied up with our thoughts, feelings, words, and actions, that it would be unwise if not impossible to give a simple definition. However, one quality is present in all people who enjoy good mental health, and that is emotional security.

People who enjoy good mental health are our neighbours; they are the postman, the workman, the typist, the executive—people who are reasonably happy, and who have the ability to get along with their families, friends, and workmates.

These members of our society have occasions when they feel unhappy, or have fits of the blues, quarrel, lose their tempers and are not themselves, but can, and do, adjust themselves to their problems, to take the ups and downs of life, the troubles, annoyances, and frustrations of daily living, and can face physical, mental, and emotional crises quite successfully. Overall, they are people who are relatively free of worry, of hate, and of anxiety.

By developing good mental health we can keep our balance, which means tolerance, understanding, compassion, making decisions, accepting responsibilities, facing up to the problems of life, and enjoying its blessings.

Good mental health has always been associated with a happy childhood. The way a child is brought up and the kind of home life he enjoys are the important factors in the moulding of the future adult. The essentials are simple: love, affection, praise and encouragement, and healthy discipline. These lead to emotional security and development of the child.

The prevention of mental ill health and the promotion of good mental health involve cultivating attitudes favourable to personal contentment, satisfaction, well-being, and an inner feeling of ease and of comfort. Such attitudes may well include the following:—

1. Being interested in the needs and welfare of others.
2. Cultivating good aims. Aim to:
   Spend and save wisely.
   Recreate and relax well.
   Help others.
   Be sociable and friendly.
   Avoid expecting too much from other people.
   Appreciate that the world is full of potential friends and interesting possibilities.
   Cultivate optimism, and be interested in things outside oneself.

A mentally healthy adult may be described as an emotionally secure, industrious, and sociable optimist with good aims.

THE HUMAN MIND
(THE STUDY OF WHICH IS CALLED PSYCHOLOGY)

No one is yet clear what the human mind looks like. As far as we know it is shapeless. And as it cannot be appreciated either physically or chemically, it has to be accepted and appreciated in the abstract. As this is an exceptionally difficult thing to do, it is far easier to imagine it as having shape and form if it is to be understood at all (*Fig.* 1). The mind can be looked upon as having four main divisions:—

The conscious division (EGO), through which we become aware of ourselves and of our surroundings.

The subconscious division, where useful memories are stored.

The unconscious (ID), which stores unpleasant memories and painful experiences. This part of the mind is not in any way

	Super-ego	
Unconscious (id)	Conscious (ego)	
	Subconscious	

Fig. 1.—Diagram of the human mind.

stagnant. It is continuously active, even when we are asleep. It is this part of the mind which accounts for our dreams and nightmares. It can, unknowingly to us, affect our conscious attitudes and standards of judgement, and is invariably at the root of symptoms associated with mental illness.

The authority principle of the mind (SUPER-EGO) sets a standard to which the ego has to conform.

In general the human mind may be looked upon as a system of images, images formed from the sensations fed to it from the various special senses. It can also be described as an adjustive system, because, without the mind and the awareness which it creates, it would be impossible to adjust intelligently to the environment and to ourselves. As a system, it may be looked upon as the eleventh system of the body.

No one knows where or what is the actual link between the mind and the brain. All we know is that the mind is dependent upon the brain. Destroy the brain and you destroy the mind with it. It is, therefore, accepted that the mind is situated in the brain.

The conscious mind (the ego) may be described as a continuous stream of changing experiences and of interacting concepts and ideas. (A concept being a meaningful image and an idea its function or use; e.g., the mental picture which we have of a fountain pen is a concept, whilst the use which we associate with it is the idea.)

The conscious mind creates thought through the processes of thinking and imagination. Thought is, therefore, the content of consciousness. Thinking, a dominant process of consciousness, has three aspects to it, and these are:—

    i. Knowing (cognition).

    ii. Doing (conation).

    iii. Feeling (affect).

In health all three function simultaneously and interact harmoniously. For as we think and become aware of a particular thing we also feel in a certain way about it and act accordingly. The type of thought which is constructed and entertained in consciousness has to conform to two standards, both of which are quite separate from the standard of authority already referred to as the super-ego. These two standards are:—

Self-esteem (a person's opinion of how clever, etc., he is).

Self-respect (the person's opinion of how good he is).

Both these standards may be considered together as *self-regard*.

Actions reflect the activity of the mind, and directly reflect what is being thought of and what has been decided upon in consciousness at that time.

Morale of a person reflects his self-esteem, and if the person is to remain optimistic and in sound mental health, self-esteem has to be well preserved. Any threat to self-esteem is a direct threat to mental health. It is therefore necessary to protect this self-esteem, especially against inferiority. The mind does this through a number of mental mechanisms, of which rationalization is one example. A poor workman who blames his tools may be doing just this.

Esteem may also be affected by conflicting forces competing for dominance, and these may exist consciously in the conscious part of the mind, or unconsciously in the unconscious part.

Failure to resolve conflict often results in mental ill health. The mind, which interacts continuously with the body, does so harmoniously in good health, but when there is lack of harmony, mental ill health results. The mind, in being active, is naturally energetic, and it derives its psychic energy from its many psychological needs, of which there are four basic ones:—

    i. Affection.
    ii. Recognition.
    iii. Security.
    iv. Responsibility.

Without needs the mind would be inactive.

MENTAL MECHANISMS

These are defences of the mind. They serve to lessen insecurity and protect self-esteem. The greater the insecurity, the greater the defence. Examples are:—

Projection

This is the basis of all forms of hallucinations and delusions. It is a mechanism by which personal faults, weaknesses, etc., are attributed to other people and to things outside ourselves. We fail to recognize these as part of us.

Reaction Formation

Reacting to a situation with an attitude which is opposite to that in the unconscious. Pity as against cruelty; humbleness as against aggression; superiority as against inferiority, etc. This may also be observed in the extreme humility of a number of epileptics and in the aggressive hatred of the paranoid.

Projection with Reaction Formation

As seen in the grand magnanimous individual who finds fault, or in the critical self-righteousness of another.

Rationalization

An apparently plausible excuse to justify an unconventional act.

Transference

Directing a sentiment to something or someone else other than the original. It is to attach such sentiments as love or hate to a substitute. We may either love or hate someone because they unconsciously remind us of someone else.

Displacement

Taking one's feeling out on some harmless object. Patient may displace aggression, hostility, violence, or any other emotion in this way.

Sublimation

Expressing basic urges in a socially acceptable way, e.g., channelling aggression into boxing, wrestling, etc. Sublimating fantasy through art and music. Learning to argue and to discuss sensibly instead of resorting to violence to prove one's point.

Fractional Repression

This results in slips of the tongue, or in thought blockage and certain forms of amnesia.

Over-compensation

Developing a skill or an attribute at the expense of all else. To bury oneself in a hobby or some other pursuit. This is invariably an attempt to overcome inferiority. Exhibitionism and excessive indulgences are often examples of over-compensation.

Other Mechanisms include:—

Disarming the critic through belittling oneself.

Seeking reflected glory by identifying oneself with someone whom we deem has greater prestige.

Belittling others.

Turning a blind eye to a painful situation, either by avoiding or refusing to talk about a particular subject, or by changing a subject abruptly in the course of a conversation. Even young children are skilful at doing this.

GROUP DYNAMICS AND PSYCHOPATHOLOGY

Group dynamics are the social and psychological forces which determine behaviour and influence interpersonal relationships.

Events, experiences, needs, wants, appetites, wishes, and desires are all involved, and by studying these we set out to explain motives, reasons, and psychopathology.

Psychopathology is the study of events and experiences and the reactions and responses which these produce in the individual. Events may involve needs, frustrations, deprivations, sufferings, and all the experiences and relationships imaginable, whilst the reactions to the events which occur within the mind may involve mental mechanisms and feelings of all sorts.

Responses are the actions or the symptoms which reflect the mental reactions. Suspicion, sullenness, aggression, timidity, stubbornness, hostility are only a few of such responses.

Psychopathology from the Freudian psychoanalytic point of view is said to involve an interplay between the ego, the super-ego, the id, and reality (or the world around us and life in general). In this respect a mental illness and its symptoms may be looked upon as a form of compromise which satisfies the ego, the super-ego, and the id. These three, as you will remember, are three of the four divisions of the mind and are integral parts of the personality.

The ego itself is expected to satisfy the demands of the super-ego and the id and the demands of the real world (reality). Normality depends upon the ego's ability to harmonize these demands whilst retaining its own identity and integrity. If the ego is unable to establish this harmony, conflicts may occur between the super-ego, id, and reality. When a conflict between the id and reality occurs, the ego may side with either one of the two.

Psychopathological Conflicts

1. Ego plus Id against Reality

Complete neglect of the demands of the real world with modification of its appearance by means of delusions and hallucinations. Reality is falsified to satisfy the ego and to grant freedom to the basic impulses of the id, though the personality still refuses to recognize the basic impulses as part of itself—probably because it still has to satisfy the demands of the super-ego. Projection is a common mechanism evolving from this.

2. Ego plus Reality against the Id

Excessive repression as observed in neuroses. Anxiety with its attendant evils develop.

3. CONFLICT BETWEEN THE EGO AND THE SUPER-EGO

May either result in:—

a. Complete dominance by the super-ego. As this crushes the ego, it results in depression with guilt feeling.

b. Complete freedom of the ego. The ego is now able to express itself freely. It becomes elated and results in mania.

MENTAL ILLNESS GIVES SATISFACTION

The development of symptoms in mental illness is a process by which the id, super-ego, and ego are all satisfied.

1. It gives expression to the id.

2. It inflicts punishment on the super-ego.

3. It may gratify the ego so far as the illness affords an easy excuse for shelving temporarily all personal responsibility.

PERSONALITY

Is a person as a whole.

Popularly described as a person standing among his fellows, and described as pleasant or unpleasant.

Personality may be viewed as having three main divisions, and these are:—

1. Disposition

A person's psychological make-up, which incorporates:—

a. Attitude

A readiness to accept or reject.

b. Basic personality

In terms of maturity, immaturity, intolerance, and insecurity. (*See* Special Duties and Skills of a Psychiatric Nurse (9), p. 68.)

c. Temperament

A person's emotional responsiveness, or susceptibility to experience a dominant emotional response.

2. Character

An acquired aspect of the personality.

The good or bad side of a person's nature.

The moral attribute which determines conduct.

3. Constitution

The physical make-up.

The factors which contribute to the moulding and development of the personality include:—

1. Internal Factors

The body's functions, chemical activities, and influences of the hormones.

2. External Factors

The relationships and experiences associated with upbringing and the environment in general.

Personality is said to be strong if assertive, dynamic, independent, and commanding. But weak if it lacks drive and initiative, does not command respect, and is dependent upon others.

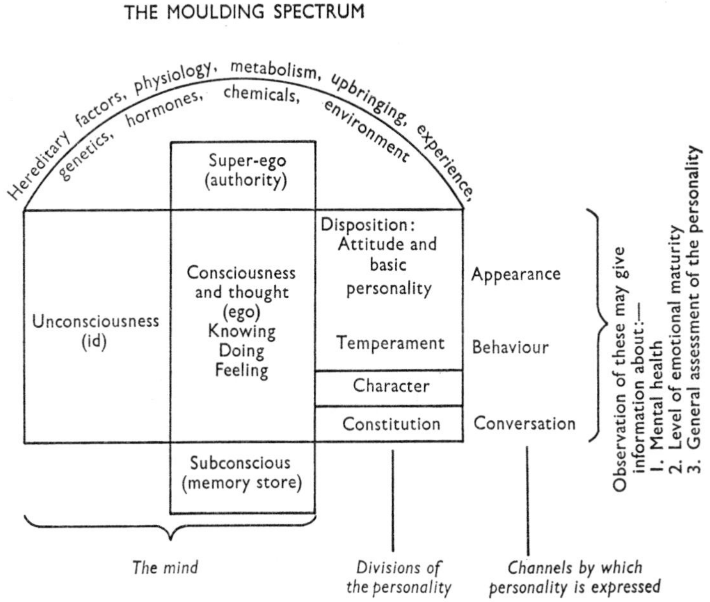

THE MOULDING SPECTRUM

Fig. 2.—Aspects of the personality as related to the mind.

An adequate personality is one which is stable physically, emotionally, intellectually, and socially.

Within social relationships, the personality may also be viewed as one having:—

a. A persona or social mask, reflected in appearance, behaviour, and conversation.

b. *The true self* of which the individual has little knowledge, but which reveals itself in attitudes and behaviour.

c. *The ego ideal* or the person's opinion of himself—his self-esteem.

d. *The opinion which others have of him.*

e. *What he considers is the opinion held by others.*

BRIEF DEFINITIONS OF BASIC PSYCHOLOGICAL TERMS

Feeling: The range between pleasantness and unpleasantness.

Emotion: A feeling of varying intensity, e.g., joy, delight, affection, anxiety, excitement, and anger.

Passion: A strong or intense emotion of a short duration, e.g., passion of anger or of affection.

Mood: The emotion prevailing over a varying period of time, lasting hours or days, e.g., elation and depression.

Sentiment: An emotional attitude composed of a cluster of emotions related to a particular object, e.g., love and hate.

Temperament: Emotional responsiveness. The way in which the emotions are expressed and experienced over a long period of time. Our susceptibility to emotional stimulation, e.g., anxious, excitable, aggressive, phlegmatic.

Orientation: To orientate is to take one's bearings. Finding one's direction.

Attitude: A readiness to act in a predetermined way; a readiness to accept or to reject.

Intelligence: All-round mental efficiency. An inborn capacity that enables us to benefit from experience, to detect absurdities, and to demonstrate foresight and creativeness.

Delusion: A false belief which is impervious to argument.

Hallucination: Perception in the absence of an external stimulus.

Confusion: Muddled thought.

Repression: An unconscious act by which painful ideas, or ideas which conflict with self-esteem, are pushed out of consciousness. Mental mechanisms serve as 'safety valves' for repression.

Obsessional Pattern: Unvaried repetitive pattern with or without insight.

Obsession: A recurring idea in consciousness over which a person has no control.

Compulsion: A compelling will-power which forces a person to perform an action.

Stereotype: Automatic, fixed, monotonous, unvaried, repetitive activity or movement.

Rumination: Constant repetitive recollection of past experiences.

Perseveration: Continuous preoccupation with, and repetition of, experiences or anticipated experiences.

Verbigeration: Continuous, purposeless repetition of words and phrases.

Fear: A violent crippling emotion.

Anxiety: An inner feeling of uneasiness associated with the fear of danger and specific functional disturbances, e.g., a fast pulse-rate.
A fear of our own nervousness.
A mild degree of fear experienced whenever a situation is seen, either consciously or unconsciously, as a direct threat to personal security and self-esteem.
A fear experienced when the individual is away from the object or thing producing it.
Nature's warning.
Alerts the body to defence through activating the autonomic nervous system.
Apprehension is anxiety in relation to an anticipated event or experience.

NEUROSES

A neurosis is an emotional disturbance. This accompanies a psychological conflict—a struggle within the mind. May be viewed as an exaggeration of what a normal person feels.

It disables in that it prevents the individual from carrying on with his or her normal working life.

Such a person persistently fails to adjust to what becomes to seem increasingly intolerable. The more he tries to adjust the worse it gets. The neurotic person is often tense and anxious, and tries without success to overcome his personal difficulties. He realises that he is not quite right; seeks advice and treatment.

Tends to make trivial complaints, though to him they are important and often urgent. Is prone to find faults with others or with the environment. Grossly insecure and lacking in confidence. Seeks reassurance and affection.

Conduct is good with attempt to keep up appearances. Conscious of social standards.

Tends to feel lonely and unwanted. Not hallucinated and usually not deluded. Somewhat immature emotionally. Personality well preserved and is often unduly pre-occupied with the need to keep up appearances. Personality is well preserved in that appearance, conduct, character, temperament, intelligence, and memory are relatively unaltered.

A neurosis may show itself as:—

a. A depression.

b. An obsessive/compulsive state.

c. Hypochondria. (Psychiatrists, however, are divided in their views of hypochondriasis. Some accept it as a neurotic state, whilst others view it as more a symptom than a condition. Of course hypochondriacal symptoms are common enough in a variety of mental conditions.)

d. Hysteria.

e. Anxiety.

f. Neurasthenia.

PSYCHOSES

A thought disturbance with disorder of reasoning predominating. Behaviour is unpredictable and somewhat odd.

A psychotic patient tends to live in a world of make-believe. Is hallucinated and deluded. Lacks insight and does not therefore realize that he is unwell.

Neglects responsibilities and personal appearance. One whose habits deteriorate quickly. Is often immodest and unconventional.

Is reluctant to seek advice and treatment. Needs continuous observation, and supervision, especially during the acute phase. Tends to be asocial or antisocial.

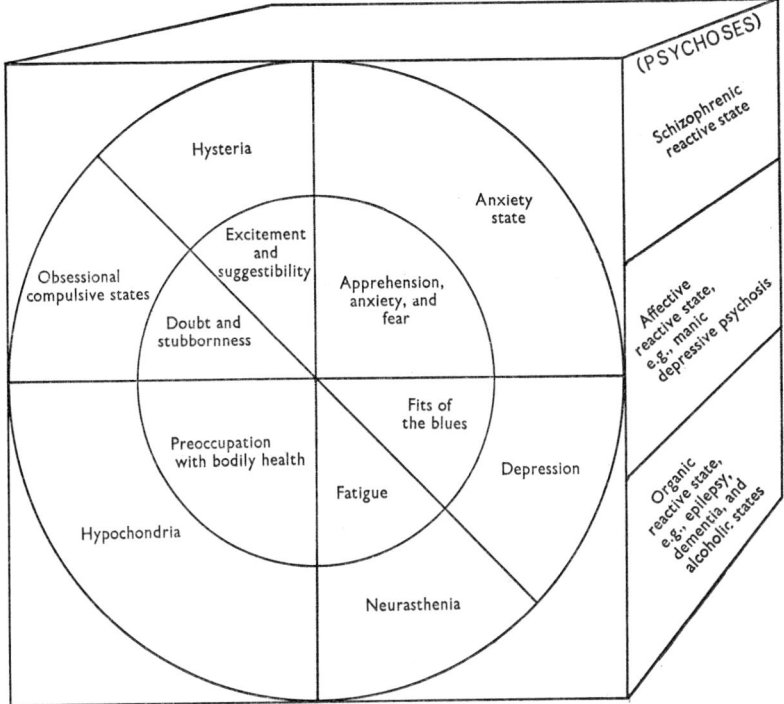

Fig. 3.—Types of mental illness in diagrammatic form. Inner ring represents the normal; outer ring, neuroses–exaggeration of the normal.

Experience and learning will show that the features dominant in particular patients vary, and that there is very rarely a typical textbook case to be seen. The above features may be taken as the ones often met with, and are not to be accepted as fixed and absolute.

SPECIAL CONSIDERATIONS IN RESPECT OF:—
Anxiety States

In an attempt to reduce anxiety and to promote confidence:—
Place the patient within a small group.

Provide with gradual increase of responsibility within the group.

Before moving the patient or altering his routine give adequate preparation.

Encourage activity which may be easily completed.

Avoid competition, especially during the acute phase.

Give work which may not be spoilt by the patient's muscular tension and sweaty hands.

Make sure that he has companionship—someone with whom he feels secure.

Hysteria

In an attempt to reduce self-display, excitement, and frustration:—

Group with patients who can accept hysterical symptoms without showing too much sympathy.

Avoid grouping with other hysterical patients.

Encourage to undertake responsibility which will gain attention in an acceptable way.

Patient should not be left on his own too long.

Divert patient's interest from symptoms through cultivating interest in current affairs and so on.

Control behaviour through changing the environment.

Encourage the patient to talk and to join small group for discussions.

Obsessional States

In an attempt to promote security and avoid undue tension:—

Have plenty of space available for the patient to work in.

Furniture, tools, and personal possessions not to be disturbed.

Avoid giving too much responsibility and expecting too high a standard.

Encourage to work obsessional pattern constructively. Select an activity which is constructive but repetitive.

Plan changes or new events well in advance.

Plan activities which are simple and which can be reached quickly.

Protect the patient from possible humiliation. It is easy to poke fun at someone who is awkward and ritualistic.

Make decisions for the patient.

Give notice of an event in plenty of time.

New tasks to be simple. Allow for repetition.

Reactive Depression

In an attempt to combat morbid introspection and social isolation without increasing anxiety:—

Group with moderately cheerful patients.

Encourage to take responsibility gradually.

Give tasks which are practical and realistic—something which they feel is going to be of value to them.

Keep active in company.

Need extra reassurance at night.

Never force into group functions. Whenever possible leave within hearing distance of group discussion. It is surprising how many do end up by joining the group by their own volition.

Change routine often, though not drastically.

Avoid monotony of routine. Introduce fresh interests daily.

Talk to the patient.

(Remember that some depressed patients can be over-active and have a 'hail fellow well met' type of behaviour.)

TYPE OF PERSON WHO MAY REQUIRE PSYCHIATRIC FIRST AID

The suicide risk.

Emotionally distressed—the grief-stricken.

Excitable and overactive.

Confused and delirious.

Fearful.

Paranoid—one who is excessively suspicious.

Psychopathic liar and exploiter.

Aggressive/noisy.

Stuporous.

One who panics.

Impulsive.

MANAGEMENT: BASIC ESSENTIALS

The Suicide Risk

Keep under observation discreetly.

Supervise unobtrusively.

Be on the look-out for a sudden change of mood.

Avoid reproach.

Reassure and persuade.

Minimize risks.

Grief-stricken

Approve of the distress experienced.
Private, quiet surroundings to allow for free expression.
Free from worry. Encourage to talk.
Secure companionship.
Reassure and persuade.
Arrange for a diversion of interest, and a change of surroundings.

Excitable and Overactive

Listen.
Persuade and reassure.
Do not restrict outlet. Channel overactivity.
Occupy.
Keep under observation.

Confused and Delirious

Do not contradict. Agree with viewpoints.
Distract. Suggest and humour (play along with the patient).
Be pleasant, kind, and tactful.
Never contemplate force. Mild restraint at times.
Keep under observation.

Fearful and Anxious

Reassure and persuade.

Paranoid

Be polite and respectful.
Avoid being overfriendly.
Interfere with as little as possible.
Observe and check unobtrusively.
Expect and be ready to accept abuse with equanimity.
Be discreet in what you do and say.
Try not to laugh and gossip in his presence.

Psychopathic Liar and Exploiter

Do not be taken in by 'crocodile' tears and bad luck stories.
Practise sceptic tolerance.
Maintain discipline.
Protect other patients.

Aggressive/Noisy

Minimize frustrations.

Look for evidence of latent aggression.
Reduce emotional tension.
Keep your distance, and do not take unnecessary risks.
Avoid undue fussiness.
Be kind but guard against being unduly generous.
Avoid conflict of wills. Be tactful.
Yield but challenge through asking what he would do in a particular circumstance.
Orders, if any, have to come from some higher authority.
Ask for his advice on certain topics.

Stuporous and Inactive

Reassure.
Talk.
Remove to a more pleasant environment.
Fuss a little.
Keep under observation.

Acute Panic Reactions

Restrain with firmness.
Promote calmness.
Reassure.
Encourage to talk: listen.
Keep under observation.
Maintain a degree of healthy discipline.

The Impulsive

On the first sign of restlessness or change of mood, investigate and increase your surveillance.

Be wary of the one who is too quiet. Give the patient some repetitive activity for short periods.

Take steps to minimize risks.

Practice due care and learn to anticipate, appreciate, and adjust to dangers with confidence, but with caution and sceptic tolerance.

Some of you may already be asking, But how, why, when, and where do I promote calmness and maintain a degree of healthy discipline, as in 'Acute panic reactions' above, for example. Unfortunately, there are no simple answers to these, and that is why I have not attempted to elaborate beyond that which has been presented.

In an emergency, the essential lies with knowing what to do quickly; there is not the time to probe much beyond this at the time. Also, it should be appreciated that the basic essentials listed above are intended only to serve as a guide to managing these various conditions. To appreciate their full practical significance, however, demands experience, learning, and practice.

When dealing with human behaviour, it is never possible to standardize responses, for no two conditions are ever alike. Also, we can never hope to follow a predetermined formula. Our approach has to vary as the situation presents itself. And the only sure way of learning how to do this successfully is through experience. There is no real substitute for this.

PRINCIPLES OF NURSING PSYCHIATRIC PATIENTS

1. Observe discreetly—and assess as you smile.

2. Supervise unobtrusively by doing things for and with the patients.

3. Practise due care, i.e., take steps to minimize risks.

4. Satisfy wants and needs casually as a matter of course.

5. Promote and protect individuality and encourage the patient to talk.

6. Get to know the patients as individuals.

7. Learn how to yield gracefully—as you yield, challenge by asking the patient what he would do in the circumstance. An occasional apology, if offered wisely, may sometimes serve to lessen aggression in a hypercritical patient.

8. Be ready to agree rather than contradict.

9. Learn to anticipate and check as a matter of routine.

10. Practise sceptic tolerance and watch as you trust. If you think the patient is unduly distrustful of you, avoid direct questioning; talk about yourself instead.

11. Reassure and persuade rather than order.

12. Be always ready to listen. Listening is often more valuable than talking.

13. Avoid reproach and the use of words with moral overtones.

14. Orders, if any, should be presented as having come from a higher authority. This is often more acceptable to the patient than if they came directly from you.

15. Minimize frustrations and boredom.

16. Learn to appreciate that patients:—

   a. Talk to relieve distress and uneasiness.

b. Find fault when they are agitated.

c. Complain to cover up embarrassment.

d. Are lively to hide shame.

e. Chat because their heads ache and they are sad.

f. Ask idle and misplaced questions when they are lonely and uncertain.

g. Show fatigue because of a reserved internal sorrow.

h. Reproach themselves when they feel guilty and anxious.

i. May be awkward and difficult because you may be difficult.

j. Over-elaborate and insist on a rigid routine because they are insecure.

k. Are excitable and over-react because they are insecure.

l. Attitude to a situation is usually more important than the situation itself.

m. Every action is an attempt to communicate.

n. However difficult they may appear, want to be friendly.

o. Are talkative, argumentative, and noisy when they are frightened.

p. Test reactions when they are insecure.

q. May be either aggressive, sullen, sulky, stubborn, or argumentative when frustrated.

17. Take care that you do not search for sincerity by studying the patient's face too much or you may make the patient unduly suspicious.

18. Avoid undue fussiness and setting too high a standard.

19. On the first sign of restlessness or change of mood be more watchful.

20. Learn through experience to adjust to dangers with caution and confidence.

21. Remember that it is an offence to ill-treat, to neglect, and to restrain a mentally sick person.

BASIC RULES IN RHYME

Manage well, or be in hell; there the devil takes the hindmost.

Check, or by heck, get it in the neck.

Make a date to anticipate.

Sanction less the moral indiscretions and fear less the aggressive inclinations.

Still waters run deep. So remember that the silent mute is not easily duped.

Stitch in time saves nine.

When life is a bit hectic, be tolerant though sceptic.

As you fight the good fight with all thy might (in being conscientious), accept the bark as worse than the bite.

EMOTIONAL TENSION

Emotional tension is captivated or pent-up feeling, which is not allowed expression either because one is afraid to express it, or because one is under the assumption that to control or bottle up feeling is a form of moral righteousness, and is therefore the correct thing to do at all times—a typical puritanical outlook.

A person who is emotionally tense is invariably awkward, both in behaviour and posture, and is often moody, irritable, and suffering from a variety of unpleasant feelings, of which indigestion, constipation, headaches, back pain, and insomnia are only a few. These are symptoms brought about by the increased muscle tone produced by the emotional tension, and are *symptoms common to neurosis and psychosomasis*.

Most people who become emotionally tense are not always aware of this, even though they may realize that something is out of place. To suggest emotional tension as a cause, however, may incite hostility and defiance, and is one way of losing friends unless made with a good deal of tact and diplomacy.

It seems much easier to blame other people and situations for the way one feels, than to accept the cause as being within oneself.

Strange as it may seem, however, most people are able to recognize frustration easily enough, and believe with conviction that they are able to detect emotional tension in others with ease and facility. But, when it comes to recognizing this in themselves, it is a different matter altogether. Perhaps this is a defence against fear and deep-seated inferiority.

Not only is emotional tension associated with increased muscle tone, but it is also associated with increased muscle tension and instability of that branch of the nervous system—the autonomic—which normally maintains a healthy activity within the various organs of the body.

Increased muscle tension is noticeable in the forceful impulsive handshake, in the ungainly posture, in the strained facial expressions, in facial tics and mannerisms; whilst instability of the autonomic nervous system produces among other things dilated pupils and a bounding pulse.

In a nutshell, emotional tension and its associated experiences are unpleasant, and give rise to much distress and unhappiness.

Suggestions on the Prevention and Relief of Emotional Tension

Some patients may benefit from being encouraged to:—

Cultivate a hobby and to seek satisfaction in helping others.

Appreciate that it is not always possible to excel in all things.

Adopt the philosophy, that, 'if once I fail, I will not give up trying, and if I am finally defeated, I will accept this with good grace, realizing that though I may be weak in this one thing, I may be strong in another'.

Cultivate the art of 'give and take', of being a host and a guest, and both a leader and a subordinate.

Learn how to accept criticism as criticism and not as opposition, and to avoid too much self-pity.

Avoid the habit of testing other people's motives and sincerity; instead, to accept people for what they are, and to appreciate that at bottom most people want to be friendly.

Set out to please others, and not to feel unduly hurt if frustrated.

Recognize and accept such feelings as jealousy and hate as quite normal. The essential thing is to be able to control these sensibly.

Talk and express viewpoints freely, but naturally with some polite reservations.

Participate in recreational pursuits to cultivate fresh interests and to expend energy. Sports of all kinds are useful here.

Relax tense muscles by taking a hot bath and if possible to undergo a course in relaxation.

Act out what a particular piece of music may conjure up or portray within his mind. And whilst he may find this awkward at first, especially as he will be required to do it with others, he will soon learn to enjoy it once he gets over his self-consciousness.

Indulge occasionally in a spate of repetitive activity, something different from the general run of things. Even doodling would help.

Seek help if situations become unbearable, and learn how to share his troubles. Two heads are better than one.

Take his prescribed drugs conscientiously.

In the final analysis, the fundamental essential in preventing and relieving emotional tension is *satisfaction of the four basic psychological needs*—security, affection, recognition, and responsibility. Failure to do this brings on emotional tension and, whilst it may not always be possible to abolish the psychological conflict which must inevitably occur at times in all of us, it is possible to release the feeling which this generates.

PSYCHOSOMATIC ILLNESSES

'Psychosomatic' simply means mind over body. The mind affects the body and its functions in an abnormal way. Illnesses of this form, and the personality types associated with them, may include:—

Rheumatism

Sociable and friendly. Neurotic traits common—fear of suffocation, nervousness and nightmares. Admire people who treat them badly.

Articular Rheumatism

Irritable and hostile, especially to any form of domineering. Emotionally unresponsive. Unpopular with associates.

Asthma (Illness of Longing)

Cling to mother. Afraid of losing mother and of being rejected by her. Expected to exercise self-control in emotional matters at an early age.

Gastric Ulcers

Desire for petting and fussing, but this is consciously denied. Longing to be dependent. Low maturity.

Coronary Insufficiency

Industrious. Ambitious. Conscientious, with a considerable amount of self-control. Fail to find proper sexual satisfaction in their marital relationship.

Heart Neurosis

Of an obsessional disposition and emotionally insecure. Friendly, obliging, and well-liked.

SOME COMPARISONS BETWEEN PSYCHOSOMASIS, NEUROSIS, AND PSYCHOGENESIS

PSYCHOSOMASIS	NEUROSIS	PSYCHOGENESIS (e.g., HYSTERIA)
Emotional disturbance secondary to physical symptoms Physical symptoms may be viewed as a substitute for an unconscious mental attitude The emotional disturbance is an indication that the person is disturbed about the physical symptoms	Emotional disturbance appears first Physical symptoms follow and are due to increased muscle tone associated with emotional tension and disturbance of the autonomic nervous system	Emotional disturbance is incidental and when it appears it is superficial and associated with excitability
Emotional reactions may be associated with anger, resentment, contempt, anxiety, worry, and fear, and a desire for consolation	Emotional reaction may be associated with fear, anxiety, doubt, and depression	Emotional reaction may arise from anger and self-pity
The cause of the condition is in the first instance outside the person's control, but once he becomes aware of his attitude, symptoms improve Condition not modified by changes in the immediate environment	The condition is completely outside the person's control and change of attitude very rarely helps Condition not modified by changes in the immediate environment	Change of attitude is reflected immediately in change of symptoms and symptoms are greatly modified by change in the environment
Body symptoms are dominant	Mental symptoms are dominant	Both mental and body symptoms often co-exist
A result of frustration	A product of psychological conflict	Associated with lack of sympathy and attention
Prognosis very favourable if seen early enough	Prognosis favourable	Prognosis unfavourable

Anxiously avoid open hostility. Dislike being alone.
Inhibited and depressed even with intimates.
Always sleep with window open.
Overdo hygienic precautions.
Heavy smokers. Drink a lot of coffee.

Migraine

Suppress anger. Lack humour. Irritable. Intellectually ambitious. Tend to be domineering as well as to take offence easily.
Jealous.

Constipation (common in three-quarters of all people who suffer from paranoia)

Pessimistic and swing towards depression. Dependent and believe that they are having a raw deal.
Sensitive to lack of generosity on part of loved one.

Diarrhoea

Feel defeated. Always feeling tired.

THE ART OF LISTENING

Listening demands interest, concentration, and understanding.
Listening requires that we attend and observe.
Some people are by nature good listeners, others are not so good.
Becoming a good listener demands that the person must learn to become interested in the subject or matter, and often interested in a person or persons.
Setting out to please others reflects a matured attitude, and is an invaluable step towards directing and controlling personal behaviour as essentials to sustained attention and interest. In other words, it all makes for poise, charm, and self-discipline, all of which are practical assets.
Self-forgetfulness also contributes to becoming a good listener, for it helps me to realize that it is not what I myself say that is important, but what the other person is saying or wants to say.
A good listener knows how to adjust to the situation, and is able through the appropriate expressions and reactions to convey an impression of sincerity, friendliness, and sympathy.
Accepting the other person as interesting is one step towards adopting an alert, eager, and friendly attitude.

Listening to a person who can be seen and who perhaps is facing us in person is essentially different from listening to a person who cannot be seen or who is seen only on a television screen, for when the person is there with us we become more concerned with him as a whole. Mannerisms and expressions become more distracting, and can interfere with concentration on what is being said.

It is an advantage to look at the person as he speaks and advisable not to gaze too much on one specific area of the person, for this can make for embarrassment and annoyance. The better way is to shift the gaze continuously but casually. Of course, a lot depends upon the attitude of the speaker to you and also upon the speaker's emotional security, for these may lessen or increase his sensitivity to your presence.

Listening helps the nurse in many ways. It encourages the patient to respect the nurse. It offers the patient opportunity to talk to someone who demonstrates sympathy and understanding. It helps the nurse to find out about certain problems of the patient.

Listening helps to reassure a worried patient, a person who just wants to talk out his worries.

Listening makes for good fellowship and is a therapeutic tool in more senses than one.

Listening is indeed a skill.

Listening requires:—

Patience and tolerance.
Self-discipline and poise.
Interest and respect.
Sympathy and equality.
Understanding and a desire to help.
Sincerity and self-forgetfulness.

SUGGESTION AND THE USE OF SUGGESTION

Success means a great deal to most of us, and in the attempt to avoid failure, we become only too eager to take advice from people whom we respect, like, and admire. This is especially apparent when in need of help, encouragement, and support, for we take advice and counsel willingly without much criticism and with little if any reasoning at the time. We become suggestible to ideas and actions of others. We often imitate and follow these blindly without questioning; it is only later that their significance may become apparent. People are by nature suggestible, some more than others, and as there are degrees of suggestibility according to the level of emotional maturity and security of the individual, it is often difficult to speculate on the outcome of any pre-arranged plan for the use of suggestion. It is often a better plan to work things out cautiously by trial and error.

A suggestion may be described as an idea transferred from one person to another, or from the environment to a person, and the acceptance of the idea without being aware of any definite reason for doing so.

There are many forms of suggestion, each with its peculiar appeal and directed to one or more of the special senses, and anyone who has watched a T.V. commercial or read a glossy magazine is well aware of this.

For general purposes, suggestion may be considered as being of three kinds:—

1. Direct.
2. Semi-direct.
3. Indirect.

1. Direct Suggestion

This takes the form of a request, the granting of a permission, or advice.

EXAMPLES

Would you like to take your hat off? (request).
You may take your hat off if you wish (permission).
You would benefit from taking your hat off (advice).

This form of suggestion is most useful with the *emotionally immature and the emotionally dependent* type of person.

2. Semi-direct Suggestion

With this form of suggestion, we link ourselves with the person, and we use the pronoun, you and/or I.

EXAMPLES

If I were you, I would take your hat off.
It would please them, if we were to take our hats off.
I wonder if you and I could put our hats somewhere.
Let's take our hats off.

This is a useful form with a person who is *in need of company, sympathy, and attention.*

3. Indirect Suggestion

Either the third person such as he, him, they, or an object or a thing is used.

EXAMPLES

He was accepted more readily by taking his hat off. (Such a statement is made casually in the presence of the person whom you think would benefit by taking his hat off.)

My brother is always a gentleman, for he never forgets to take his hat off when entering someone else's house.

The indirect form of suggestion is useful with the *potentially hostile, intolerant, suspicious, and aggressive type of person.*

Suggestion forms an essential part of persuasion with suggestion as the part which appeals to our pride and esteem.

The first basic step in the use of suggestion is to find out what the person wants, and to realize that most people would secretly like to have a bargain or to have something for nothing, and perhaps to have an excuse for making merry. So by offering an opportunity for these, with the chance for the person to prove himself, to become accepted and to be liked, loved, and admired, he may be made more susceptible to suggestion. This is a practical, constructive, positive approach to creating a disposition favourable to suggestion.

In the event of hostility being encountered in the use of suggestion, it is always wise to apologize immediately, to give reasons why the suggestion was made, to remain calm, composed, and patient at all costs, and to ask the person for his opinion on the matter in hand. By adopting this course it would be possible to retain the initiative and to prevent loss of face, and always avoid giving the person the impression that you are embarrassed, frightened, annoyed, or guilty, lest it might increase aggression and make the person uncomfortably bossy and domineering.

Whenever suggestion is being used there is always a need for caution, and a need to guard against becoming smug, superior in manner, and talking down to the person, even though we may be tempted to do this when we notice how gullible and credulous some people can be at times. Suggestibility, if in the extreme, renders the individual less able to express his individuality, assertion, and independence, and can in this respect be a severe handicap. Such persons need our protection.

There are other people who demonstrate a high degree of contra-suggestibility in that they automatically do the opposite to what is being suggested. It is an advantage to be aware of this, for positive use can be be made of it in appropriate circumstances, e.g., telling a person to keep his hat on may incite him to take it off, and if this is what we wanted him to do in the first instance, we would have made positive use of this peculiar response.

Suggestion used wisely can be an effective therapeutic tool, and always of immense value to a nurse. Are we always aware of its practicability and importance? Perhaps we should attempt to become a little more suggestion-wise.

BLOCK ANALYSIS OF PRACTICAL PSYCHOTHERAPEUTIC TECHNIQUES

Reassurance

To restore confidence.

ORDER OF APPROACH AND PROCEDURE

a. Establish physical contact. The traditional handshake might possibly be the method of choice in this respect, or perhaps placing the hand casually on the shoulder might help. However, if touching, do so with caution, because some patients may resent this.

Giving and sharing, though constituting a less direct approach, may be quite effective, because as one hands over something to someone else, the bridge made is indirectly a way of making physical contact.

b. Establish equality. One way of doing this would be to adopt a position similar to that taken up by the patient, e.g., if the patient is sitting down, then sit down yourself, etc.

c. Build confidence. Emphasize the positive like saying 'do' rather than 'don't'. By accepting how the person feels and sympathizing accordingly, it is possible to establish a friendly relationship.

Encourage the patient to talk, and listen intently with compassion and sincerity. Find something to praise, and use your powers of persuasion to point out the advantages and disadvantages of a certain line of thought or of action.

d. Promote personal comfort.

e. Create a diversion of interest by encouraging the patient to help someone else, and perhaps to indulge in some repetitive activity for a short time. This would help to reduce emotional tension.

f. Build up a pleasant atmosphere and combat loneliness at all times. If possible never leave alone too long in the early stages.

Persuasion
ORDER OF APPROACH AND PROCEDURE

a. Agree with and approve aspects of what the patient believes in or is doing.

b. Build confidence in the manner suggested above under Reassurance.

c. Suggest an alternative to what the patient is preoccupied with, and imply that you only expect its acceptance for a short period.

Point out the advantages of doing this to the patient.

Remain calm and patient at all costs. Never raise your voice in anger if you feel you are not getting anywhere.

Appeal to the patient's self-esteem and personal regard, and the possible effect of his attitude upon other people, especially upon friends and those dear to him.

Pursue this line of approach diligently.

d. Next leave for a short time to think things over.

e. In about half an hour or so, return and ask if he has come to any decision.

f. As a last resort imply disapproval and disinterest in a casual nonchalant way. And whilst this approach might hurt his pride a little, it should not in any way have a lasting detrimental effect upon the relationship between the nurse and the patient. Much, of course, depends upon how skilful the nurse is in doing this. If she does it with sincerity and respect, there should be little to worry about.

g. Be tactful, and practise due care throughout.

As you reassure and persuade do so with kindness, pleasantness, patience, sincerity, and confidence. Also, take your time to promote a relationship and an atmosphere based upon informality with respect, and upon equality with responsibility.

SUGGESTIONS ON HOW TO DIRECT CONVERSATION TO FIND THE MENTAL STATE OF A PATIENT

In the field of psychiatry, it is often very difficult to define clearly the demarcation between areas of activities and interests of respective clinical and social workers. Definite areas, however, do exist; for there are many contrasting responsibilities.

The main difference between each participant, however, whether it be a social worker, nurse, or psychiatrist, seems to be more with the area of activity and interest of each than with the persons themselves.

The psychiatrist differs from a nurse in that he is required to diagnose and prescribe treatment, whilst the nurse is expected to supervise and therefore to manage people in various situations. The overall care, however, is a combined responsibility of both, and this is the common ground on which they can meet as partners.

What, it may be asked, does the nurse assess when she attempts to find out something about the mental state of a patient? Does this differ from what the psychiatrist assesses? The answer is, of course, yes.

The nurse is predominantly concerned with the attitudes of patients to given situations, and with their ability and capacity to manage situations as they arise. The psychiatrist is more concerned with assessing the patient's potentiality in relation to future events. What a psychiatrist may now conceive as a future event, however, may quite easily be the nurse's immediate concern in the 'present, tomorrow'. Present situations and patient's reactions to these are always a major concern of a nurse.

The psychiatrist's interest, of course, enters into the area of activity of a nurse, but his main preoccupation is usually with analysing and assessing personalities, understanding psychopathology, and evaluating the nature and degree of incapacity. The range of interest and concern are indeed wide, and covering such subjects as those presented below in the form of a mnemonic.

The mnemonic is URAMI PACT SIN COD.

In general, the nurse is more concerned with the PACT SIN COD than with the URAMI. Her knowledge of URAMI should be as practical as possible.

Mnemonic Explained

U   Unconscious forces—complexes.
R   Reasoning.
A   Attention.
M   Memory and mental mechanisms.
I   Intelligence.

P   Preoccupations—what the person keeps on thinking about.
A   Attitudes, especially to the environment and to people.
C⎫ Conversational Themes—what the person talks about. Is
T⎭ there a repetitive theme underlying what is being said?
    Knowledge of this would help the nurse and the psychia-
    trist to know about the basic problems of the patient. A
    repetitive theme reveals preoccupation with worries, doubts,
    and allied states.

S   Suggestibility.
I   Interests.
N   Needs.

C   Contact with reality.
O   Orientation.
D   Distractability.

Direct questions are best avoided by the nurse unless it is
desirable to ask about personal health and comfort; things that we
all seem to talk about pretty easily. 'How are you feeling these
days?' it may be asked. 'Is your health improving?'; 'Have you
managed to see the doctor yet?'; 'Are you being looked after
well?'; 'Is there anything you want?'; 'Do you sleep well, or are
you like me, going to sleep in a chair early evening and finding that
I cannot sleep when I get to bed, or if I drop off to sleep, I
invariably wake up early morning?'; 'Here is the newspaper for
you to look at'; 'Would you like me to get you some library
books? What sort would you like me to get?'

Replies to such an assortment of questions and statements may
reveal immediate interest, basic need, dominant attitudes, and
immediate problems. Some patients may talk freely about themselves and their experience, and often without much prompting;
others, however, may be more cautious and uncommunicative.
With the suspicious and the guarded, a more indirect approach is
always best. They could be encouraged to comment on things in
general through the medium of a general conversation.

On meeting a new patient, one could start by saying 'So you are Mr. Jackson, an ex-policeman. How are you?' Responses may show whether or not the patient realizes who he is, and how he accepts the approach. Is he relaxed or tense, suspicious or trustful, aggressive or timid.

'Haven't the years gone quickly', it may be said in an attempt to find if the person is appreciative of, or is orientated to, time. 'Where do you think I come from?' you may ask. 'I'll give you three guesses. I think I know where you come from. Would you like me to guess? Don't the years go by quickly?' 'Yes, they certainly do, and how things have changed. I suppose most people hanker after the so-called 'good old days'. Personally, I get a certain amount of pleasure and satisfaction in recollecting memories from my early years, although I suppose it is healthier to think of what it's going to be like in the future.' Answers or comments may reveal attitude, memory, insight, optimism, volition, and orientation.

Direct remarks about people, unless they are complimentary, are best avoided. It is usually safer to limit comments about people to how good, kind, or clever they are. This makes for more trust.

'Did you see that programme on the T.V. last night? What a lot of rubbish it was.' 'I believe it's time they painted this room.' 'Isn't it different since they painted this room?' 'Yes, it is a much more pleasant ward now.'

The above is intended to give some idea on how to direct conversation, though it is not planned to follow any definite pattern. The idea is to make it as natural and as spontaneous as possible whilst still testing reactions, and exploring attitudes, interests, needs, orientation, suggestibility, and distractibility.

This is a mere guide, and whilst interpretation of responses will unavoidably be speculative, they will nevertheless be pointers to further observations and understanding.

It is essential as always to keep an open mind, to avoid hasty decisions, to be willing and ready to modify assumptions, and to refrain from passing moral judgement on what a person may view as fault or weakness in others. The aim of a nurse as always is to help the patient in every way possible, and that is the object of this approach, for through wise handling of a conversation much can be learnt about the problems of others and of the best way to help them.

DELUSIONS

A delusion is a false belief.

Impervious to reason, argument, and education.

Not in keeping with the general belief of either the community, society, or race to which the individual belongs.

Dominates thinking.

(How does a delusion differ from a superstition ?)

Main Types of Delusions

1. GRANDEUR
Saturated with self-importance and of feeling personal superiority. Self-esteem is inflated out of all proportion.

2. UNWORTHINESS
Believes that he is inferior, inadequate, and unfit to live. He may, in his own estimation, be an unpardonable sinner.

May also believe that he is bringing disgrace on others.

Whole mood is dominated by guilt.

3. HYPOCHONDRIACAL
Believes that in one way or another he is diseased.

4. PERSECUTORY
Believes that people and situations are against him. Sensitive and suspicious.

5. NIHILISTIC
Believes that nothing exists, or that everything is dead.

Some of the Problems associated with Delusions in General

Lack of concentration due to the intense preoccupation with the delusion.

Misinterpretation of information and of other people's motives.

Impulsive and aggressive outbursts resulting in violence.

Awkwardness of behaviour which embarrasses and which possibly annoys others.

Sullenness, stubbornness, and reluctance to co-operate.

HALLUCINATIONS

An hallucination is a disorder of perception.

Often described as perception in the absence of an external stimulus.

It is not always easy to decide on whether or not a person is hallucinated, because much depends upon observation and on what the patient says. It is not always easy to be certain of the facts.

Example

Because a patient is talking to the wall, it could be assumed that he is hallucinated, whilst, in actual fact, he is either talking to himself, or indirectly to you by the aid of the wall. He is possibly too self-conscious and timid to shower you with abuse directly.

Most hallucinations have a *delusional component* in the sense that the *patient believes* that he is sensing things.

Hallucinations involve the special senses, and for convenience may be classed as follows:—

1. *Auditory*: Voices and sounds are heard.

2. *Visual*: Things are seen.

3. *Olfactory*: Smells of all kinds may be experienced.

4. *Gustatory*: Involves taste.

5. *Cutaneous*: Involves skin sensations in general.

6. *Hypnogogic*: An hallucination involving any of the special senses, and experienced often by many normal people when half awake.

The general problems associated with hallucinations are similar to those listed for delusions.

CONSIDERATIONS ON SCHIZOPHRENIA

Schizophrenia is a psychosis occurring in a number of young people of the shut-in type of personality. Up to the present there is no known specific cause for this, although much is speculated, and a great deal of research is involved. Schizophrenia is sometimes referred to as a 'split mind', and accounts for about 40 per cent of patients in psychiatric hospitals.

The *symptoms* of schizophrenia are of two types—those like depression, tension, and difficulty in concentration, which occur in other forms of mental illness, and those peculiar to schizophrenia and which are disturbances of thinking, of emotion, of will-power, and of movement. It is also characterized by special forms of delusions and hallucinations.

(*See* mnemonics, p. 97).

Suggestions on the Management of the Acute Phase of Schizophrenia

Give the patient large uncomplicated repetitive projects with a minimum of colour. Colours, however, may be bright, but too many tend to confuse the patient.

Give simple commands such as 'let us take a walk'.

At first, try not to offer a choice, lest it might incite aggression.

If correction is necessary, do it quietly by saying 'do it this way'.

Try not to tell the patient he is doing wrong, because as he is highly sensitive to criticism he may either become discouraged and withdraw into his shell, or become confused, erratic, and hostile.

In general he is very sensitive to his inadequacies and to scorn.

He needs constant reassurance about his dress, behaviour, and so on, and requires encouragement to take pride in his appearance and standard of general cleanliness.

This type of patient avoids people, and more than two people in a room can be most irritating.

On the whole he appreciates someone talking to him, because this helps to bring him out of his dream world. Care, however, is required to avoid breaking suddenly into his fantasies. Anticipate impulsive actions at all times.

As this condition is associated with delusions, hallucinations, and fragmentation of thought, the world outside is distorted and this is one reason why he seems so awkward. Much patience, tact, and skill are therefore required to secure some measure of co-operation.

The nurse who cares for this type of patient needs to be a skilful observer, well versed in the skills of management. What he needs above all else is the service of a calm cool-headed friend, someone who is able to take a genuine interest in him as a person.

There are four main types of schizophrenia—the paranoid, the catatonic, the hebephrenic, and the simple. (*See* a standard textbook of psychiatry for details, and refer to the mnemonics on p. 97 of this handbook.)

Principles in the Management of the Paranoid Type

By the way, being paranoid implies that a person is suspicious, feels persecuted, and is lacking in insight.

Suspicion by itself is quite a normal trait. It is only when it is associated with persecution that it becomes abnormal.

Give this type of patient time to size up a situation.

Realize that he is cautious and does not rush into anything.

Avoid over-friendliness and allow good relationships to develop gradually.

Avoid competitive situations, because competition only increases suspicion and distrust. Give opportunity to excel without having to compete with others.

Recognize and meet the patient on his own intellectual level, and divert interest from delusions, rather than trying to oppose them.

Permit and encourage graded responsibility, especially in organizing things, e.g., cataloguing library, organizing dances, clubs, and committees. But do not be over-eager to appoint this person a chairman of a committee. He is usually much too hostile, aggressive, and intolerant for this.

Remember that he works best on his own, and, whenever possible, encourage him to externalize aggression in some useful pursuit, e.g., gardening. Appreciate that you and others are under critical observation all the time. It is therefore unwise to hold private conversations in his presence.

Try to give direct answers to questions.

Correspondence may have to be checked especially if it is liable to be abusive and condemnatory.

Realize that his dominant need is recognition.

Be on the look-out for this patient's subtle influence on other patients.

Appreciate that he is usually intelligent, critical, intolerant, adept at creating sympathy, eager to dominate, highly independent, ambitious, uncompromising, and grand.

Much skill and experience is therefore required to manage this rather awkward person effectively. The management of this type of patient should not be left to the inexperienced.

PRINCIPLES OF NURSING AFFECTIVE STATES

Examples of these are melancholia and mania. These make up what is often called cyclothymia—a 'mood-swinging' illness, with two phases to it, depression and elation.

Appreciate the value of routine, covering a 24-hour schedule. This promotes security, protection, and discipline.

Build up a satisfactory nurse–patient relationship, and as soon as the patient is well enough, introduce into the climate of a therapeutic community (*see* p. 94).

Always be on the look-out for a sudden change in outlook and behaviour, especially as this may be a manifestation of 'reaction formation' (*see* Mental Mechanisms, p. 29). Examples of this manifestation would be a patient who up to a particular period was restless, but who became suddenly calm and composed, or the reserved patient becoming talkative and over-active. Extra vigilance is therefore required when this occurs, for, who knows, they may imply a more deep-seated intent. The first example might suggest that suicide is contemplated, whilst the second may suggest violence.

Specific Nursing Considerations in Respect of the Depressive Phase—Endogenous Depression, Melancholia

Place patient with others; avoid keeping in isolation.

Introduce to group activities gradually.

Externalize guilt through getting the patient to perform a service for other people.

In the early stages make decisions for him.

Give time for the patient to follow what you are saying, and do not rush things.

Keep under distant observation unless actively suicidal.

Avoid treating as a child. Realize that he is fully rational, and quite possibly of good intelligence.

Take steps to avoid fatigue.

Keep from draughts and away from impulsive patients.

POSSIBLE COMPLICATIONS

Suicide.

Loss of weight.

Secondary infection, e.g., pneumonia.

Dehydration and malnutrition.

Self-mutilation, e.g., picking the skin and pulling hair out.

Constipation.

Retention of urine.

Guilt is believed to be a fundamental issue in endogenous depression, and it is responsible, apparently, for the self-reproach and remorse so characteristic of this illness.

However, guilt may also be experienced by many other people as well.

Reactions to guilt are numerous, and here are a few examples.
A person may become:—

Apathetic and depressed.

Preoccupied, restless, and sleepless.

Aggressive and blaming others.

Increasingly generous, without apparent reason.

Over-anxious about the welfare of someone close to him.

Self-conscious, embarrassed, and blushing.

Over-active and hard working.

Apologetic and making frequent excuses over a particular
incident.

Over-friendly, over-active, with a 'hail fellow well met' type of
attitude.

There are other possible reasons for this kind of response. What
is needed is experience and intelligence to single out the most
probable cause or reason for such response. Perhaps the most
fundamental essential is to accept awkward and odd responses with
sceptic tolerance and without undue criticism.

MANIA

There are four main types:—

Hypomania: Producing restless, over-active, interfering busy-
bodies.

Acute mania: Producing a wild, frenzied, aggressive attack of
excitement and over-activity.

Chronic mania: Sometimes called Scott's mania.

Hypermania: Delirious or Bell's mania.

Three dominant features of mania are restlessness, excitement,
and over-activity. Mania is associated with the more extroverted
type of personality. (Refer to a standard textbook of psychiatry
for more detail of symptoms.)

Principles of Management

At first, place the patient on his own in a quiet environment.

Externalize aggression as soon as possible in some out-of-door
pursuit, but allow for adequate rest to prevent exhaustion.

As the patient becomes less over-active, introduce to controlled
rhythmical movement. Perhaps a little dancing might help, as long
as you do not expect too much expertise. Reduce irritating and
frustrating influences, and avoid long conversations. Never imply

threat or punishment or you may incite violence. Also, avoid arguments and discussions.

Make full use of his distractibility and suggestibility, although do not expect too much consistency, because he is bound to be highly erratic and without much tenacity.

Correct and adjust the environment rather than the patient— a calm atmosphere tends to calm the patient, whilst a noisy one excites.

It may also help to control the range of colours in his immediate environment. Never be tempted to make fun of the patient.

Possible Complications

Violence.

Exhaustion.

Malnutrition.

Dehydration.

Heart failure.

Secondary infection.

NURSING THE DEMENTED, THE MENTALLY SUBNORMAL, OR THE MENTALLY AND PHYSICALLY DETERIORATED

First it may be necessary to train good habits—habits in respect of cleanliness, toilet, feeding.

Once these have been cultivated it may then be possible to consider training in respect of SHOCS:—

Self Help and independence.

Occupation and the acquisition of a useful skill.

Communication.

Socialization.

Principles of Socialization

1. To establish and maintain a planned programme of group functions.

2. To encourage patients to organize the programme themselves.

3. Nurses to mix in with patients, and to advise when necessary or when asked.

4. Routine to be organized to meet patients' needs.

5. To foster trust and a spirit of service within a climate of acceptance and appreciation.

6. To maintain an atmosphere of activity, interest, and enthusiasm.

DEMENTIA AND SUBNORMALITY

Dementia

Deterioration of intelligence.

Subnormality of Intelligence

Lack of intelligence from birth or from an early age.

All forms of training require routine with plenty of repetition.

Tasks to be of a simple nature to start off with.

All tasks however simple should be broken down to their simplest forms to allow for some measure of understanding.

ASSESSING PATIENT'S PROGRESS IN SOCIAL RELATIONSHIPS

Consider degrees of social responsiveness:—

Conduct—modesty, reserve, and respect.

Interest.

Confidence.

Self-regard.

Pleasure.

Satisfaction.

Awareness of people.

Friendliness.

Social abilities in respect of acting as hosts or hostesses.

Personal appearance.

Imitation of others.

Appreciate that most patients within this category are slow, dependent, lacking in insight and foresight, and prone to accidents and neglect. Their nursing may come within that of graded nursing care, i.e., according to the degree of progress and of deterioration.

PSYCHOPATHY

Classed as a mental disorder rather than a mental illness.

In the Mental Health Act 1959 psychopathy is defined as 'A persistent disorder or disability of mind (whether or not including

subnormality of intelligence) which results in abnormally aggressive or seriously irresponsible conduct on the part of the patient,
and requires or is susceptible to medical treatment'.

Some Specific Comparisons between an Hysterical Personality and a Psychopathic Type of the more Aggressive Form

HYSTERICAL	AGGRESSIVE PSYCHOPATH
On the whole respects authority	Anti-authoritarian, rebellious, and derives thrills and pleasure out of being 'naughty and anti-social'
Seeks sympathy, and sympathy tends to exaggerate the condition	Seeks recognition and wants to be dominant
Immature by nature, and seeks pleasantness	Intolerant disposition
Does not particularly exploit people and situations. Is a manipulator more than an exploiter*	Exploits people and situations
Can tolerate frustration	Cannot tolerate frustrations
Over-reacts impulsively with exaggerated responses and exhibitionism. Puts on airs and graces—being over-sophisticated	Exhibitionistic chiefly—anti-conventional
Suggestible; mood varies with the tone of the environment	Contra-suggestible—tends to do the opposite to what is asked. Mood influenced by personal attitude at the time
Regrets wrong-doing	Lacks regret in wrong-doing
Character is good usually	Character invariably defective
Emotionally unstable	Socially and emotionally unstable
Excitable	Plausible and boastful
Functional symptoms common, e.g., fits	Physical symptoms rare

* A manipulator makes use of people and situations, whilst an exploiter not
only makes use of people and situations, but may also take what belongs to other
people, especially if there is a reasonable chance of getting away with it.

Dominant Features

May be described as a disorder of conduct and of character with the following features:—

On the whole a psychopath resents authority, is rebellious, and cannot stand frustrations.

He is a person who derives thrills out of committing anti-social acts, and does not respect the feelings of others.

Other features which exist, but which are displayed with less consistency and predictably perhaps than the foregoing are:—

A psychopath is egocentric, immature, and demands his own way 'by hook or by crook'. He is generally irresponsible, lacks self-discipline, and is intolerant. Though of good intelligence he fails to learn from experience.

He is usually plausible and very skilful at exploiting others, a trait well recognized in a confidence trickster. In general (and unless being dependable, etc., is a means to personal gain) he can be unreliable, undependable, unpredictable, and disloyal to the extreme.

Types of Psychopathy

THE AGGRESSIVE

A predominantly anti-social type, with destructive inclinations.

THE INADEQUATE

The emotionally dependent, credulous, lying, and passive type who may drift into crime.

THE CREATIVE

The eccentric, flamboyant, and passionate type, whose perverted interests may bring on disrepute.

Principles of Nursing Psychopaths

As they resent authority and cannot put up with frustrations, it is advisable to keep frustrations to a minimum if at all possible and to maintain discipline on a group basis. Encourage the group to make rules and to approve rewards, sanctions, and penalties.

It may be advisable to segregate from other types of mental disorders in an attempt to protect other patients from exploitation.

In your assessment of these patients be objective, factual, and noncommittal. Always remember that a harmless statement made in innocence can be elaborated and exaggerated out of all proportion. Never get involved in an argument and be firm without losing your temper. Maintain activity and work effort. Also, always check and assess the work completed. It is essential for discipline to maintain a fairly high standard of work and efficiency. Be consistent and fair in your attitude and approach, and cultivate the art of persuasion. Privileges are allowed, but only on the basis of give and take. One gives only if it is reciprocated in another way. This must be one of the standard rules. Maintain a routine, and expect the patient to conform to this, and whenever possible to appreciate the situation in terms of 'we'. Beyond this, encouragement is given to each individual to express his individuality and to use his initiative in a way acceptable to the majority.

The word *delinquent* is sometimes used to describe a person who persistently acts without regard for others.

BASIC PRINCIPLES OF CARE OF AGGRESSIVE/ SUICIDAL PATIENTS

1. Supervise unobtrusively.

2. Try to find the cause and deal with this if possible.

3. Speculate on what might be the immediate need of the patient.

4. Appreciate that actions, however awkward they may be, communicate, and that aggression/suicidal attempt is an appeal for help.

5. Attend to the environment and to the tone of the social atmosphere. Often a noisy atmosphere precipitates noise, whilst a quiet one does the opposite.

6. Consider the effect which this disturbance may have on other patients and on the staff. Speculate on whether or not it might engender hostility, restlessness, discontentment, self-reproach, scapegoating, and so on.

Aggression

1. A driving force associated with a wish to dominate a situation.

2. Intentionally asserting oneself to harm another person, or to damage something.

Violence

An aggressive physical force, directed towards a situation.

SPECIAL DUTIES AND SKILLS OF A PSYCHIATRIC NURSE

1. Appreciates and deals with group situations.

2. Analyses problems relative to the situations in which they are found. Problems are therefore situational.

3. Interprets situations and relationships objectively. Looks for reasons and causes other than intentions, and attempts to see situations as they really exist.

4. Interprets problems and situations *without moralizing*, and avoids the use of words having negative moralizing overtones, e.g., inferiority, average, escape.

5. Considers and appreciates the *opposites of exaggerated social responses*. Prefers not to take things at their face value.

6. Appreciates that often the attitude to a situation is more important than the situation itself.

7. Appreciates that every *action* is an attempt to *communicate*.

8. Helps patients as people to adjust to a way of life compatible with their background and social standing: assists with re-motivation.

9. Appreciates the influence of basic personalities on relationships and situations, e.g., the immature personality which seeks excitement, thrills, and pleasantness, the intolerant personality which seeks faults, the insecure personality which seeks sincerity and security.

10. Appreciates that fundamentally every person, however difficult and awkward they may appear, wants to be *friendly*.

11. Knows how best to deal with awkward emotional attachments and transference.

12. Is skilled in the art of *reassurance and persuasion*: appreciates the subtlety of human behaviour.

13. Is aware of the influence which the nurse's presentation has on the reactions of patients, e.g., a patient may be awkward because the nurse is awkward, and vice versa.

14. Supervises patients unobtrusively with tact and understanding of situations and relationships in depth.

Supervision involves being skilful in the art of:—

Observation.
Anticipation.
Checking.
Recording.
Reporting.

Establishing satisfactory nurse–patient relationships.
Satisfying needs of patients.
Promoting well-being, comfort, and morale.
Taking all necessary steps to protect the patients.
Caring for each patient conscientiously.
Persuasion, reassurance, and the use of suggestion.
A psychiatric nurse may be viewed as a nurse and a therapist. As a therapist she satisfies needs through managing behaviour and situations, whilst as a nurse she satisfies needs and provides care in an attempt to make situations and relationships pleasant and acceptable.

CAUSES OF MENTAL ILLNESS

MNEMONIC

HEADS or TAILS

H Heredity.
Hereditary.

T Toxins, drugs, chemicals.
Trauma (injury).

E Endocrine.
Environment.
Exposure to extreme
  climatic conditions.

A Alcohol, apoplexy, age.

A Accidents.

I Impregnation—pregnancy.

D Deprivation of love, food,
  oxygen, etc.
Disease (physical), e.g.,
  heart failure.
Deterioration of the brain.

L Loss of a faculty: blindness, deafness,
  lameness, paralysis.

S Stress (social), e.g.,
  bereavement, financial
  difficulties, emotional
  deprivation.

S Syphilis—a venereal disease
  which may damage the
  nervous system.

Cause may also be considered as:—

Predisposing

That which favours or is favourable to the breakdown from the start, e.g., a constitutional weakness, being hypersensitive and a worrier.

Precipitating

That which hastens the breakdown, or which increases a person's susceptibility, e.g., repeated failures.

Exciting

That which by direct action or impact starts the illness, e.g., financial collapse—the last straw which broke the camel's back, so to speak.

A combination of factors such as these could quite likely produce a severe bout of depression.

BRIEF OUTLINE OF TREATMENTS USED IN PSYCHIATRY

1. Drugs

a. TRANQUILLIZERS, e.g., Largactil (chloropromazine) (calm and clear consciousness of delusions and hallucinations, Melleril (thioridazine), Serenace (haloperidol), Valium (diazepam) (reduces tension and anxiety).

b. ANTI-DEPRESSANTS, e.g., Tryptizol (amitryptyline), Tofranil (imipramine).

c. ANTI-CONVULSANTS, e.g., Luminal (phenobarbitone), Epanutin (phenytoin sodium), Valium. These prevent and reduce epileptic fits.

d. STIMULANTS, e.g., benzedrine, which is amphetamine—contained in 'purple hearts'.

e. HYPNOTICS, e.g., non-barbiturates such as Mogadon (nitrazepan) and Mandrax (methaqualone), and barbiturates—common one used is sodium amytal.

f. ANALGESICS (pain relievers), e.g., codeine and aspirin.

A sedative is a drug which calms, relieves pain, and produces sleep. Morphine and pethedine would be in this category.

2. Electro–convulsive Therapy (E.C.T.)

Mainly used in depression.

3. Modified Insulin

Used for anxiety states, drug addiction, and alcoholism. Stimulates appetite as well.

4. Narcosis

Deep sleep treatment. Patient is kept asleep for the largest part of 24 hours (up to 22 hours). This treatment lasts for about 14 days. Used for drug addicts and alcoholics.

5. Neurosurgery

Relieves chronic depression, obsessions, and compulsions. It also reduces aggression.

6. Psychotherapy

This involves persuasion and reassurance with or without hypnosis. Group discussions. Art and music appreciation. Play reading. Acting out to music. Use of suggestion.

7. Behaviour Therapy

To correct faulty behaviour and to overcome morbid fears (phobias). Aversion therapy is included here. Aversion therapy is generally used for the treatment of sexual deviations and alcoholism.

8. Occupational Therapy

A creative activity performed at leisure and which aims at keeping patients active and creatively employed.

VALUES OF THIS TREATMENT

Overcomes boredom.
Promotes sociability.
Resocializes.
Boosts morale.
Combats introspection.
Satisfies curiosity.
Relieves emotional tension.
Keeps the patient active.

9. Vitamin Therapy

Fatigue and confusion, especially in elderly patients, may be associated with vitamin deficiency, so the administration of vitamins serves to correct this.

10. Hormonal Therapy

As hormonal imbalance may give rise to mental symptoms, it becomes necessary to correct this by the administration of one or more of the hormones concerned.

GROUPS OF DRUGS USED IN THE TREATMENT OF PSYCHIATRIC ILLNESS

1. Ataractic Drugs

These clear consciousness of confusion, delusions, and hallucinations, and are otherwise known as major tranquillizers.

a. Phenothiazines

Largactil (chlorpromazine).
Stelazine (trifluoperazine).
Sparine (promazine).
Pacatal (mepazine).
Moditen (fluphenazine) and Modecate (fluphenazine decanoate). Both the latter are long-acting injectable forms of phenothiazine. They are injected intramuscularly. Absorption is gradual over a number of weeks. Most useful in the rehabilitation of long-stay schizophrenics.

b. Serenace (haloperidol)

(Lithium carbonate is a non-phenothiazine drug used in the treatment of mania.)

2. Anti-depressants

a. Tofranil (imipramine)

b. Monoamine Oxidase Inhibitors. These block the release of the monoamine oxidase enzyme in the brain. Examples: Parnate (tranylcypromine), Nardil (phenelzine), Marplan (isocarboxazid).

The administration of this group of drugs may give rise to hypertension resulting in severe headaches, and death or permanent brain damage from cerebral haemorrhage. Patients on these drugs should avoid eating cheese, Bovril, and Marmite.

c. Tryptizol (amitriptyline).

3. The Emotional Tranquillizers

The minor tranquillizers, e.g., Librium (chlordiazepoxide), Equanil and Miltown (meprobamate), Valium (diazepam).

4. Hypnotics

Barbiturates.
Doriden (glutethimide).
Indorm (propiomazine).
Mandrax (methaqualone).
Chloral hydrate.
Paraldehyde.

5. Analeptics

These counteract narcosis, e.g., picrotoxin, leptazol, Megimide (bemegride).

6. Central Nervous System Stimulants

These produce prolonged stimulation, e.g., amphetamine as contained in Drinamyl and Mylodex (dexamphetamine sulphate), Meratran (pripradrol).

7. Anti-convulsants

Luminal (phenobarbitone).
Phenurone (phenacemide).
The hydantoin group of drugs, e.g., Epanutin (phenytoin sodium).
Valium (diazepam).

8. Psychomimetic Drugs

These mimic psychoses, e.g., Mescaline and lysergic acid (L.S.D.).

9. Anti-Parkinsonism

E.g., Artane (benzhexol), Cogentin (benztropine), Disipal (orphenadrine).

10. Anabolizers

Bodybuilders, e.g., Durabolin (nandrolone).

11. Vitamins

12. Hormones

13. Anti-histamines

E.g., Benadryl (diphenhydramine), Antistin (antazoline), Anthisan (mepyramine). These counteract allergic reactions.

VITAMIN THERAPY

The B-complex group is the most commonly used.

Lack of vitamin B_1 may result in depression, feeling of lassitude, irritability, difficulty of concentration, anxiety, and diminished mental acuity.

TRANQUILLIZERS

Approved Name	Trade Name	Average Daily Dose	Principal Side-effects	Toxic Effects
Chlorpromazine	Largactil	75 mg.	Drowsiness Hypotension Parkinsonism	Jaundice Blood abnormalities Photosensitivity
Promazine	Sparine	75 mg.	Hypotension Tremors	Blood abnormalities
Acepromazine	Notensil	30 mg.	Hypotension	—
Prochlorperazine	Stemetil Compazine	15 mg.	Parkinsonism Restlessness	—
Trifluorperazine	Stelazine	10 mg.	Drowsiness Parkinsonism Restlessness	—
Perphenazine	Fentazin Trilafon	6 mg.	Dystonic reactions are frequent, e.g., facial grimacing and facial distortions, and stiffness of neck	—
Pecazine	Pacatal	75 mg.	Drowsiness Parkinsonism	Agranulocytosis—a condition due to the absence or reduction in the number of granulocytes— polymorphonuclear cells. This results in pyrexia, and ulceration of the throat Jaundice

TRANQUILLIZERS—*continued*

APPROVED NAME	TRADE NAME	AVERAGE DAILY DOSE	PRINCIPAL SIDE-EFFECTS	TOXIC EFFECTS
Thioridazine	Melleril	75 mg.	Minimal side-effects	—
Reserpine	Serpasil	8–12 mg.	Severe depression Fall in body-temperature Low blood-pressure Salivation Parkinsonism	—
Haloperidol	Serenace	2–15 mg.	Motor restlessness (akathisia) Parkinsonism Dystonic reactions	—
Thioproperazine	Majeptil	Up to 90 mg.	Parkinsonism Dystonic reactions Sweating Salivation	—
Fluphenazine	Moditen and Modecate Prolixin	25 mg. 120 mg.	Restlessness and tremors Hypotension Paraesthesia	— —

ANTI-DEPRESSANTS

Approved Name	Trade Name	Average Daily Dose	Principal Side-effects	Toxic Effects
Iproniazid	Marsilid	75–150 mg.	Hypomania Hypotension Oedema Schizophrenic symptoms may become worse	Fatal liver necrosis
Phenelzine	Nardil	45 mg.	Oedema Hypotension Nausea	—
Nialimide	Niamid	25–150 mg.	Dry mouth Sweating Dizziness Blurred vision	—
Isocarboxazid	Marplan	30 mg.	Coryza-like symptoms Oedema Hypotension	Hepatitis has been reported
Pheniprazine	Cavodil	Up to 12 mg.	Hypotension Constipation Blurred vision Dry mouth	To be used with caution in patients with liver dysfunction

ANTI-DEPRESSANTS—*continued*

APPROVED NAME	TRADE NAME	AVERAGE DAILY DOSE	PRINCIPAL SIDE-EFFECTS	TOXIC EFFECTS
Imipramine	Tofranil	Up to 300 mg.	Dry mouth Oedema Pruritus Hypotension	—
Amitriptyline	Tryptizol	100 mg.	Dizziness Dry mouth Nausea Paraesthesia of limbs (pins and needles) Drowsiness	—
Tranylcypromine	Parnate	30 mg.	Restlessness Dizziness Dry mouth	—

The most common anxiolytic drug in common use is diazepam (Valium), average daily dose being 4–40 mg. in divided doses. The most common side-effect is drowsiness. Headaches, hypotension, and impaired speech may also occur. Toxic effects are similar to those for tranquillizers in general.

Early Symptoms of Nicotinic Acid Deficiency

Lassitude, apprehension, depression, amnesia, disorientation, confusion, hysteria, and maniacal outbursts.

Lack of vitamins A and D may cause night terrors in children. Vitamin C and nicotinic acid are given in confusional states.

HORMONAL TREATMENT

Mental stability is related to endocrine function. In myxoedema there may be confusion, neurasthenic symptoms, states of depression, and anxiety with or without a paranoid aspect.

Menopausal symptoms may be treated by oestrin. Symptoms include anxiety and paranoid ideas, or rapidly fluctuating mood changes.

Premenstrual tension states are characterized by mental tension, irritability, depression, insomnia. Treated by progesterone or testosterone preparation.

Some of the neurotic and psychotic manifestations of the puerperium are helped by progesterone.

Stilboestrol has been used in the treatment of obsessional states and schizophrenia where prolonged tension states with an overflow along sexual channels takes place. Aggressive psychopaths and sexual psychopaths may also benefit by the administration of stilboestrol.

ELECTROPLEXY (ELECTRO-CONVULSIVE THERAPY— E.C.T.)

This treatment is assumed to be concerned with disrupting and altering the existing brain pattern and exciting the lower cerebral centres—the hypothalmus and the medulla.

Von Meduna, a Hungarian, observed that epilepsy was less frequent in patients suffering from schizophrenia and so he thought that epilepsy was antagonistic to schizophrenia. From this idea originated convulsive therapy. The first substance used was camphor in oil. The use of electricity was suggested by Cerletti, an Italian.

Electro-convulsive therapy may be given bilaterally or unilaterally. There is an advantage in giving it to one side of the head (unilaterally); it produces less confusion and memory impairment than when applied to both sides of the head (bilaterally). In the unilateral method, electrodes are applied to the temperoparietal region of the skull over the non-dominant side of the brain. The general procedure may be considered under the following headings:—

1. Selection of the patients by the doctor.
2. Preparation of the patient, the bed, the trolley with its accessories by the nurse.
3. The actual treatment.
4. Aftercare.

E.C.T. may be indicated in schizophrenia, involutional depression, manic states with confusion, neurotic depression, conversional hysteria when there is paralysis, but not in anxiety hysteria. E.C.T. in any form is contra-indicated in cardiac failure, following coronary occlusion, in severe lung conditions, and within six months of leucotomy.

Modified E.C.T.

This is the method of today. It is E.C.T. with the use of an anaesthetic and a muscle relaxant. This prevents the severe muscular contractions which would otherwise occur and which could result in a fracture.

PROCEDURE BEFOREHAND

Some patients will need reassuring, for it is only natural to be a little apprehensive. No food to be given for at least 4 hours before treatment.

Atropine sulphate 1/50–1/100 gr. (1·2–0·6 mg.) given subcutaneously into the superficial part of the muscle about ½-hour beforehand.

Dentures to be removed.

Bladder emptied.

Tight clothing to be loosened and shoes removed.

Patient lies on a protected bed or treatment couch.

SEQUENCE OF TREATMENT

Anaesthetic is administered. A sleep dose of sodium thiopentone or methohexitone sodium (Brietal). Some anaesthetists prefer to give the atropine intravenously at this stage.

This is followed by the administration of a suitable muscle relaxant intravenously. Methonium compounds of which scoline and Brevidil E (suxemethonium bromide) are examples of those in general use.

Oxygen inhalation may be given next.

Mouth gag is then inserted.

Shock is given.

Airway is inserted.

Oxygen under positive hand pressure is given until the effect of the muscle relaxant has worked off.

The patient is then taken into the recovery area and kept under close observation.

A sucker, an aspirating machine, and an oxygen resuscitator have to be standing by.

The nurse has to watch the patient's colour, breathing, and pulse. Complications following modified E.C.T. are very rare. The most common is impairment of intelligence and memory for a short period afterwards. Full recovery occurs in 3–4 weeks.

Pneumonia and heart failure can occur in the elderly.

The Ectonus Type of E.C.T.

This method reduces the need for relaxants and anaesthetics.

Here the current is increased rapidly from 0 to 150 volts. This takes place in about 2 seconds. The quick increase produces instantaneous loss of consciousness.

Schizophrenics require a rapid increase in 1 or 2 seconds.

Depressives require a slower increase—2–4 seconds.

Twitching is almost absent with this method.

Headache, which some patients may complain of after E.C.T., may be treated by aspirin.

A course of E.C.T. improves appetite and improves the capacity for sleep. Colour is improved and there is renewed energy and interest in life.

MODIFIED INSULIN

Given to co-operative patients whose physical health has deteriorated.

Depression, drug addiction, anxiety, hypochondria, are all conditions treated by modified insulin.

Treatment lasts 3–6 weeks.

Object is to produce hypoglycaemia. Start with insulin soluble, dose 5–10 units.

Treatment for the day is interrupted at about 10 a.m. Patient drinks a cup full of glucose.

Patients put on weight and as the result of this they look and feel better for it. This is apart from the effect of the treatment itself.

Some patients have resistance against insulin, and before coma is reached, large doses of insulin have to be given. Sometimes it is possible to overcome this by changing the brand of insulin. It is now believed that some patients possess antibodies against insulin, and that is why resistance takes place.

CONTINUOUS NARCOSIS

This is a continuous sleep treatment.

Drugs like Mandrax, Largactil, barbiturates—Dial (allobarbitone), Somnifaine, sodium amytal—are given at intervals to produce sleep.

The object is to allay excitement and anxiety. Suggestions can be made when the patient is drowsy.

Procedures may be considered under the following headings:—

1. Selection of patients.

2. Preparation of the patient psychologically and physically.

3. Preparation of a room. This to be warm, well ventilated, easily darkened, and accessible.

4. Procedure of commencing treatment. Attention during treatment.

5. Aftercare.

Preparation of the Patient

Psychiatrist explains the object of the treatment.

Patient is bathed, weighed, administered an enema, passes urine, dentures removed, changes into pyjamas.

Bed to be low, protected, and warm. In the early stages, the patient may choose the number of pillows he needs.

Procedure

Treatment is started in the evening. The drug is administered. The room is darkened and the patient sleeps. When he wakes up he is given a drink and, if need be, his mouth is cleansed. He passes urine. More drug is given and the patient returns to sleep. Every time the patient wakes up he is attended to and given more drug. Gradually, he becomes drowsy. Greater care will now be required. The nurse gives the patient full nursing attention.

He is washed, clothes changed if necessary, bed made, pressure areas attended to, mouth cleansed, patient passes urine, enema at least twice a week. Arms and legs are exercised, nourishing fluids given, T.P.R. taken and also blood-pressure.

Pyrexia and vomiting may occur about the fifth day. This is a reaction to the drugs. Treatment is interrupted.

Charts are kept for intake and output. Time and dosage of drugs noted. Urine tested daily for albumen, ketones, and sugar.

The nurse should be on the look-out for the following complications: retention of urine; dryness of skin; rash; vomiting; pyrexia; dehydration; constipation; infected mouth; pneumonia. Convulsions may also occur.

(Important to ensure that the patient receives an adequate supply of vitamins.)

Aftercare

The drug is withdrawn gradually as the treatment ceases. The treatment lasts about 14–21 days.

The patient is exposed gradually to daylight and the presence of other people.

PSYCHOTHERAPY

This is a communicative treatment directed from one person to another. It is aimed at improving a patient's capacity to deal with his own problems, to adjust himself to the demands of the environment, and to make the best possible use of his own emotional and intellectual resources. It involves trying to alter the patient's circumstances or his immediate feelings and altering the patient's innate capacities for dealing with any circumstance. This may include solving personal conflicts.

Success depends upon having a working relationship between doctor and patient. This the doctor manages through tact, honesty, and emotional detachment. For success it is necessary for the doctor to be accepted without hostility.

Psychotherapy is mainly used in the treatment of psychosomatic complaints and neurotic disorders. The individual form of psychotherapy may be considered under three headings, namely:—

1. Initial Contact with the Patient

Includes receiving the facts of his illness and establishing a psychotherapeutic relationship. To establish this relationship requires considerable skill. Later it is the manipulation of this relationship which helps the patient. The physical condition is also considered, for the patient will respond better if he is in good physical health.

The doctor takes the personal history, obtaining knowledge about the relationships which the patient preferred, the patient's temperament traits, any environmental stresses and strains, any preoccupations and associations of the patient. After this he raises topics for discussion, then becomes passive, and merely listens to the patient. Guards against expressing any opinion or making critical comments.

2. Second Phase

This involves reassuring the patient, advising him, and interpreting his problems.

This phase develops gradually. The patient is encouraged to explore the significance of his symptoms, and to make changes in his way of living.

Sessions may be taken daily or once, twice, or thrice weekly for a number of years and may last a variable length of time. Short assertive sessions are designed to do little more than reassure.

3. End of Treatment

Interval between treatments lengthened.

Patient is encouraged to test himself by making decisions and conducting own affairs.

Gradually the interview becomes a matter of observation and not therapeutic.

Patient should now have a feeling of confidence.

Willingness to return at any time if necessary.

Sometimes there is a danger of the patient developing a chronic dependence on the therapist.

Psychotherapy may take other forms. It may take the form of group therapy where patients are selected beforehand, or group therapy where patients are selected from an open group.

Group therapy of the first kind originated during the war when there was a shortage of psychotherapists.

This therapy is analytical in nature, carried out where the atmosphere is permissive but still conventional.

Discussion is the basis. It is useful with neurotics.

Selection of patients is made on the basis of personalities.

Size of the group is not more than 10.

It can be a mixed group.

It is an ideal method for out-patients, as the contact between patients is not too continuous. It is difficult to establish it within the hospital, because of the more permanent mixing and contact which takes place between patients.

Procedure is as follows:—

Start with discussing symptoms. Symptoms will be of a sympathetic nature. Interest is aroused and group unity evolves.

Patients are encouraged to interpret each other's difficulties. Projections, reflections, and abreaction occur freely. Rationalization also occurs.

The therapist does not take an active part, but he is present and the patients are sensitive to his presence. Any antagonism towards the therapist should be interpreted immediately, or otherwise the group unity would suffer and hostility would spread.

Discussion on sex produces sexual stimulation, and this tends to neutralize sexual conflicts.

A session lasts for about $1\frac{1}{2}$ hours.

Attempt is made to have two people of similar problems or interest, e.g., same religion, two homosexuals, two married persons.

The group may or may not choose a leader.

The other form of group therapy is where patients are received without preliminary selection, although this is only the first step in a series of groups. The first group may be accepted as an open general group. A number of psychiatrists attend. Gradually, the group is split up into smaller units, with one psychiatrist in charge. Next a process of selection sets in, where patients who are not compatible with the unit and the interest of the group are eliminated.

The group remaining becomes a closed group. No one is allowed in from outside the group. Discussions are now indulged in.

Psychotherapy may also be conveniently divided into major and minor.

MAJOR

Includes psychoanalysis, narco-analysis, and abreaction under hypnosis or by the aid of drugs.

MINOR

May be divided into:—

Reassurance with a placebo and sympathetic listening.

Reassurance by education, with support and encouragement to persevere.

Simple reassurance after excluding physical disease.

Abreaction by the aid of discussions.

Abreaction=the process of releasing a repressed emotion, in other words it is an emotional release.

RELAXATION THERAPY

This form of treatment is most useful either on its own or in conjunction with psychotherapy. Its main objective is to calm the mind and to reduce emotional tension through muscle relaxation. Relaxing the body relaxes the mind and helps the patient to gain confidence and a brighter outlook on life. The importance of relaxation cannot be overstressed, for fatigue and sometimes pain accompany persistent muscle tension.

The first essential is to promote muscle awareness by getting the person to think about and to concentrate on the contraction and relaxation of groups of muscles. The usual procedure is to start with one foot and work upwards. Breathing should be quiet and easy at all times.

A patient as he lies on a bed 'gives up' his entire weight to this bed. He then stretches his arms and legs as one sometimes does on waking up in the morning. Following this, the patient is instructed to take a deep breath and to stretch all his limbs. This is repeated several times, and the patient is to imagine himself heavy.

By the time the whole body has been contracted, rested, and thought of as heavy, the average patient will be feeling quite sleepy. At this stage, the patient is encouraged to think of pleasant things, of spring and summer in the country, of favourite walks, and of birds singing in the trees.

As he becomes rested, he is encouraged to stretch his whole body as before, but this time to think of his muscles as strong and powerful. The yawn as he breathes out should be one of satisfaction.

Once this is over, the patient is then allowed to get up slowly. Treatment is given daily. And when used in conjunction with diazepam (Valium), it is amazing how quickly the patient unwinds.

THE TRANSFERENCE SITUATION

This is a situation often encountered in psychiatry, and some have even gone as far as saying that what makes psychiatric nursing unique, is the ability to encourage and to manipulate transference to the advantage of both nurse and patient. As a nurse spends more time than any other member of the hospital staff with patients she is likely to become emotionally attached to them. Transference is a situation where one person transfers a love or hate to another person. It may occur either between patients, between patients and nurses, or even between nurses and other members of the hospital staff.

A patient may do this from not having had the opportunity of becoming emotionally involved before, like the emotionally deprived child or the person who has been subjected to indifference or neglect most of his life.

At times love or hate is transferred on identifying a nurse with someone from the past, someone who may have been loathed but who nevertheless had to be respected. Such experience would not only have driven hate underground but would also have generated a tremendous amount of latent hostility and emotional tension.

In the nursing relationship, transference creates many problems. But, before referring to these problems, consider how transference affects the person involved.

Transference of Love

This shows itself in:—
The increased attention which is given the other person.
Improving personal appearance.
Showing admiration and being protective at all times.
A strong desire to possess the other person and to be close by.
A constant attempt to please unstintingly and to perform the most difficult of tasks with this in mind.

Transference of Hate

This cuts the other way.
Usually hostility, contempt, and disrespect are openly displayed, although on occasions sullenness, stubbornness, and passive resistance may be the only manifestations.

Nursing Difficulties arising from:—

1. TRANSFERENCE OF LOVE
   a. Patient ignores duties and responsibilities.

b. Nurse may find the relationship becoming over-tiring.

c. The patient may be found to be intensely jealous of rivals.

d. Patient may exhaust himself in trying to please.

e. It makes for emotional tension.

f. Patient may become moody and awkward when the nurse is absent, or if the nurse does not respond favourably.

g. The patient may be exploited easily.

h. The nurse may tell the patients things in a moment of self-pity. This she may regret later.

i. The patient may attempt to bribe the nurse in an attempt to gain affection.

2. TRANSFERENCE OF HATE

Patient may:—

a. Attempt to humiliate and abuse the nurse in the presence of others.

b. Spread malicious lies in an attempt to discredit the nurse.

c. Refuse attention and nursing care from the nurse concerned.

d. Run away from the hospital in an attempt to get away from the nurse.

e. Become aggressive and even violent towards the nurse.

Manipulating transference successfully is a skilled job requiring a considerable amount of experience, and no one should set out deliberately to promote transference unless it is approved first by the doctor in charge of the patient.

On the other hand, no one can avoid the spontaneous transference which occurs between patient and nurse. All we can hope for is that the nurse is experienced to detect this and is sensible and mature enough to avoid getting too involved emotionally.

In skilled hands, transference has a therapeutic potential.

BEHAVIOUR THERAPY

A practical form of treatment aimed at correcting purposeless, awkward, and often embarrassing actions and/or attitudes, so that the person's responses in general become sociably acceptable, compatible with personal esteem, and conducive to his well-being.

Establishing this requires that useless responses such as fear of heights, etc., are modified and substituted by useful ones.

This process of modification and substitution is usually referred to as conditioning or, in simpler words, getting used to something by repetition, familiarization, and change.

In an attempt to avoid pain, punishment, fear, and general unhealthy and unpleasant responses, conditioning goes on continuously in everyone's life. Unfortunately, however, many unhealthy and unpleasant responses appear as if out of nowhere and are usually most disturbing, detrimental to self-esteem and social relationships, and fill certain people with dismay, alarm, and sometimes fear. On the whole, however, normal people repeat the more favourable responses. Some, however, are unlucky in that circumstances force them to repeat unfavourable responses at the expense of well-being.

Methods of Treatment in General Use include:—

1. DESENSITIZATION by getting the person used to the unpleasant experience gradually. And this may occur with or without it being accompanied by a pleasant experience. (Anxiety and fear may be reduced if a pleasant stimulus accompanying it is experienced in just sufficient quantity to exceed the degree of anxiety and fear experienced.) This is called 'reciprocal inhibition'.

2. RE-ESTABLISHING POSITIVE MOTIVATION by reassurance, persuasion, and the use of rewards.

3. AVERSION: correction induced by producing an unpleasant experience either in the form of a physiological upset, e.g., sickness, or in the form of a physical discomfort, e.g., electric shocks.

Behaviour Therapy is associated with Three Types of Stimuli

1. NEED: signifies a desire to compensate or to fulfil a deficiency.

2. OPERANT: in knowing how to go about getting what a person desires. What must now be done to get it.

3. RE-INFORCEMENT: satisfaction increases desire, and will therefore incite further attempt, and repetition of a successful action.

Success invariably depends upon satisfactory motivation and a *motive* can be described as that which determines action and the direction of an individual's behaviour. It is a conative–affective factor, and an impulsion from a need.

Motivation is the operation of a motive, and the study of all factors applicable to this. Certain people are said to lack positive motivation when they are inactive, disinterested, indifferent, and reluctant to seek personal gains compatible with normal standards.

To motivate means to arouse a motive, usually by supplying an incentive in the form of a reward, pleasure, freedom from unpleasantness and pain, satisfaction of needs.

Once motivated, the demand for initiative then becomes apparent and by *initiative* is meant a spontaneous readiness to act with integrity, confidence, and deliberation, in an attempt to secure an advantage or a benefit for oneself or for others.

OCCUPATIONAL THERAPY

This indicates that the patients are occupying themselves. It is a means to an end, the end being the activity. The patients may be encouraged to construct or create as they wish. Those capable of constructive work are encouraged to make something which they feel is of interest to them. The value, however, is not in the article produced, but in the activity involved.

In organizing occupational therapy it is essential to consider the facilities, equipment, and space available, the age, sex, mental condition, dominant attitudes, special skills, social status of the patient, his ability to concentrate, and general comfort.

Procedure

Classify patients into neurotics and psychotics, of recent and late admissions. Next grade the work to the patient.

Work may range from matching and rolling up wool to basket making, rug making, soft toy making, marquetry, carpentry, model making, needlework, book binding, and painting.

Make the activity attractive. In other words, try to sell him the activity. (Make sure he is comfortable, appeal to his sense of beauty by using colours and perhaps something pleasing to the touch.)

Take it for granted that the patient does not want to do anything; in that way you will be trying to coax and to interest him. Let your manner indicate that you expect his full co-operation. Don't confuse him by asking what he wants to do. Take a chance on beginning with some task which is too simple rather than one which is too difficult.

Appreciate the psychological value of success and promote this from the outset. Praise him when he has done well, otherwise use praise discriminately. Encourage good posture and watch for signs of fatigue and of boredom. Also be concerned with seating arrangements, length of period occupied, use of incentives, tea breaks, and so on.

Habit Training

This is a training programme aimed at improving the habits of deteriorated patients.

The size of the group is best kept to about 10 patients.

Success of training will depend upon punctuality of attending to, and the maintenance of, a rigid routine, conscientiousness of the staff, constant repetition, supervision, and the use of praise, encouragement, and rewards. A 24-hour schedule is usually drawn up, and this is adhered to without fail. Gradually, as the patient improves, he is regraded and placed with a more socially orientated group of patients.

Work of a simple kind is also included in the schedule and it does not matter how repetitive this is at first; the main thing is to get the patient doing something.

REHABILITATION

This means to restore the capacity and the ability to make satisfactory social adjustments.

Rehabilitation involves three phases:—

1. Training.

2. Recreation.

3. Resocialization.

Whilst these are essential stages of rehabilitation, it does not necessarily mean that they are all applicable to every circumstance. Much depends upon the degree and type of handicap and the adaptability of the person concerned.

However, rehabilitation is overall a skilled job, requiring patience, understanding, and a genuine interest in people. On occasions it can be laborious and time-consuming, whilst on other occasions it is comparatively easy and soon completed.

In a way rehabilitation is a bridge between the stage of dependency which illness enforces and the more permanent stage of independence which a normal healthy person enjoys.

Rehabilitation is an essential part of convalescence, for as we convalesce, we rehabilitate.

The Training and Learning Aspects of Rehabilitation

TRAINING

Is the process of acquiring habits and practical skills by instruction, imitation, and repetition.

The end-product of training is mechanical learning, and this is reinforced by practice and experience.

INSTRUCTION

Is an integral part of training.

It is the active process of demonstrating the method best suited to a procedure or to a specific skill.

When instructing it is useful to assume that there is a right way —an efficient way—of doing everything.

TEACHING

Is an active process of communicating information and knowledge in the manner best suited to learning, but relative to the situation as a dynamic field of experience, in which it takes place.

A teacher has to be adaptable, accommodating, and resourceful.

Intelligent learning is the end-product of teaching.

EDUCATION

Is the complex process of increasing a person's overall capacity to make satisfactory adjustment to life in general.

Education involves training, teaching, and learning.

LEARNING

Is the process of acquiring the 'know how' and the 'know why' of an experience and of replacing old responses with new ones.

As a process by which old responses are replaced by new ones, learning can be mechanical or insightful.

Mechanical learning: This occurs by trial and error as when different movements are tried out, also by imitation, repetition, and experience and by suggestion.

Insightful learning: This involves judging a situation critically, by weighing up and evaluating its many attributes one against the other.

Laws of learning: These are factual statements concerning the specific influence of various factors on learning.

Examples:—

Degree of learning is dependent upon the level of perceptual constancy. Learning is easier and more effective when *perception* is constant. Perception is said to be constant if not unduly affected by the individual's emotions and unconscious processes and by changes in the environment.

An act which fulfils some need of the individual in the learning situation is more easily learnt.

When an act is rewarded and performed under conditions favourable to learning it is more easily performed later on.

Learning by associations require that associated events must fall within a specific time limit or as near as possible to each other.

Learning is easier when the material to be learnt is meaningful. The essential first step therefore is to make material as meaningful as possible.

The rate of learning depends upon interest and the individual's strength of response to a situation. So whatever enhances these, increases the rate of learning.

When effort is increased performance rises towards the optimum. But once optimum is reached further increase in effort results in a falling performance. It seems that everyone has a saturation point.

To sum up

Learning is more effective if:—

Things are perceived as they actually are, and not as they appear, or for what we may want them to be.

It satisfies a need.

It is associated with a reward and favourable conditions.

Events reinforce each other and are closely related in time.

The material is meaningful.

There is interest.

Effort is directed towards the optimum and not beyond it.

Psychological Problems associated with Rehabilitation

Doubt of self-value with lack of confidence.

Hurt pride. This may make the patient feel unduly sorry for himself.

Emotional tension due to suppressed anxiety, worry, and aggression.

Emotional crises when anxiety, worry, and aggression are openly displayed.

Misery and unhappiness.

Over-enthusiasm and excessive desire to succeed and to prove oneself.

Hostility and increased suspicion.

Behaviour Problems associated with Rehabilitation

May include the following:—

Over-activity and emotional over-reactions.

Impulsiveness.

Attempting too much quickly.

Over-elaboration. This means overdoing things and trying to be too perfect.

Stubbornness and truculence.

Excessive fault-finding and scapegoating.

Unco-operativeness.

Taking a Group of Long-stay Patients for a Walk or on a Shopping Expedition, etc.

A. PRIOR

1. Preparation of the patients with regard to dress and personal cleanliness. See that the patients are smart and well dressed and as normal looking as anyone else.

2. Briefing of the patients as to the objective of the outing.

3. Special instructions as to freedom of action and independence permitted.

4. Collection of any special equipment, e.g., shopping bag or handbag.

5. Planning route, destination, time, projects, catering, etc.

6. Selection of staff to accompany the patients.

7. Checking to make sure that the patients will have had their medication.

B. DURING

1. Organization and deployment of group—whenever possible allow the patients to walk in pairs or in small groups.

2. Responsibilities of the nurse. To mix with the patients and to keep a discreet check on selected patients. Make the patients feel that they are trusted.

3. Meeting the demands of the patients. Some may demand extra pocket-money.

C. AFTER

1. Submitting a report to the nurse in charge on the outcome of the outing.

2. Storing equipment, etc.

3. Resting, toileting, settling down to the ward.

4. Reflections on the value of the outing by having an informal discussion with the patients.

REFLECTIONS ON A 'THERAPEUTIC COMMUNITY'

A therapeutic community is in many respects a democratic community of a special kind. It is democratic in that it encourages free expression of speech and of action, and is concerned more with the needs of the individual than with those of the community or of the environment. Personal needs are its immediate concern, but whilst it may neglect some of these other needs at times, it does not entirely ignore them. It is special in that it is orientated to treating mentally sick people and because it is generally less totalitarian than the type of community we are used to.

It is therapeutic in that it is organized to satisfy the direct personal needs of people: personal needs have priority. It is also therapeutic in that it is constantly seeking the most effective way of promoting the well-being and emotional security of people. It reduces tension, anxiety, agitation, and aggression. It combats inferiority and indifference. It builds hope, optimism, and assertion, and lessens many compulsive rituals. It discourages dogmatism and makes the concern for conventional respectability less emphatic.

A therapeutic community is a way of life directed through community effort to preventing and overcoming apathy and inactivity, and to building trust, affection, sociability, and a healthy, tolerant view of society. It therefore has to be permissive, less dictatorial, and much less formal than many of the more usual communities. If a person wishes to stay in bed, he may do so without reproach, and if he does not wish to wear his coat or such like, he need not. It is considered wrong to force a person to do things against his will, and to make him feel guilty over not having conformed with conventional routine, like washing before breakfast, getting up at a set time, and making the bed. Attempts, however, are made to encourage the person to participate in activities that are helpful to the community. Reasons for doing this would have to be acceptable to the person concerned and not only acceptable to others. A person is encouraged to clean the floor only if he thinks it necessary. He can wash the crockery if he wants to. If he wants to drink from an unwashed cup, he may do so. It is up to the individual. Authoritative commands such as 'you must', 'you have to', and 'you musn't' are avoided. It is considered much more creative to say 'you may', 'we would like you', and 'you could do this instead'.

In a therapeutic community there is also very little concern with work output and efficiency as we know them; they are not dominant issues, although attempts are made to create awareness of work and efficiency of a kind. This is fostered through appreciating that if needs are to be satisfied it becomes necessary to work, to produce, to earn, and to supply the necessary requirements. To realize the value of personal effort is one of the first steps in learning how to live in a civilized community.

In a therapeutic community, discipline, which is normally necessary for group stability and unity, is highly flexible. As far as possible, discipline is the direct concern of the person himself. There are no definite set rules and regulations within the community to enforce discipline. Discipline exists not because authority demands it, but because the individual has a wish to conform. The community, however, may influence this wish to conform through expressing approval and disapproval. Most people are sensitive to these. Group sanctions do exist, and occasionally it becomes necessary at a community meeting for individuals to account for their actions and behaviour, especially if these happen to involve or to disturb others. Gradually, it is expected that the person concerned would learn to value working with the group, rather than against it, and in the group, rather than outside it, but naturally it is up to the individual to decide on how best to adjust. There is no dictatorial insistence on doing any of this.

Gross antisocial and destructive behaviour is dealt with as an emergency with the community agreeing, though sometimes on medical advice, to immediate authoritative action for the sole purpose of protecting the individual and others from harm, and to help the disturbed person to regain composure. Once this has been achieved, the authoritative action ceases immediately. This is one time when definite authoritative action is considered justifiable. Individuals are not necessarily penalized for wrongdoing, unless the community considers that this would have definite therapeutic value.

Activities within the community are the concern of the whole community, with each member intimately involved in all that goes on. There are no ward committees in this kind of therapeutic community, and no administrative interference from sources outside the community. The community is relatively autonomous. Outsiders may be viewed as interlopers and may only enter by invitation. All members of the community meet for discussion at least once daily, and more frequently if necessary.

A therapeutic community is not in any way a secret society. There are no swearing-in ceremonies, and no fee is charged for joining. People join because it is considered advisable for them to do this on medical grounds.

A therapeutic community demonstrates a unity of purpose in its aims to promote social and emotional security, social equality, freedom of choice, freedom of speech, freedom of action involving personal matters, personal responsibility for personal care, standards of personal cleanliness, standards of cleanliness of personal environment with its utilities—clothing, bed, books, and so forth, freedom of action in manner of dress, in choice of interest, and in the pattern of routine conducive to privacy and independence. Medical advice may, however, be necessary to decide on the extent and degree of freedom best suited to each person as an individual.

A therapeutic community gives the opportunity to challenge authority, to express individuality, and to use initiative in relaxed, persuasive, encouraging surroundings. It is a community freed of despots, tyrants, and accusing pointing fingers, and is built on love, friendship, sympathy, and understanding, with respect for human dignity and individuality.

One possible danger associated with it, however, is that it could nurture 'intolerant extroversion' with an excitable, noisy, reckless, irresponsible, and disrespectful type of behaviour, a behaviour characteristic of the undisciplined child and the emotionally immature.

Nevertheless, the advantages of a therapeutic community exceed its disadvantages, and it is at last becoming more than a mere fashionable concept; it is now an observable practical entity, and it looks as if it is here to stay. It is as a stable, active, pleasant community, involving friendly relationships between people of all kinds, that it merits support and appreciation.

AID TO LEARNING THE MOST PROMINENT FEATURES OF THE VARIOUS MENTAL CONDITIONS IN A MNEMONIC FORM

Anxiety Neurosis
Remember FAINT

F   Fear

A   Apprehension

I   Irritability

N   Nightmares

T   Tension
    Tremors

Anorexia Nervosa
Remember HOOD

H   Hysterical Features

O   Over-activity

O   Obsessional Features

D   Depression

Hysteria
Remember SNIF DAD

S   Somnambulism (sleep walking)

N   Narcolepsy (uncontrollable desire to sleep)

I   Immaturity

F   Fugues (wandering episodes during which time there is amnesia for past events)

D   Dissociation (splitting up of consciousness by material pushed into it from the unconscious. Symptoms resulting from dissociation include confusion and amnesia)

A   Automatism (involuntary actions)

D   Displacement (e.g., conversion, when a mental conflict is converted into a physical disability)

Obsessional Neurosis

Remember OT OF OI OE

OT Obsessive Thoughts

OF Obsessive Fears

OI Obsessive Impulses

OE Over Elaborations

Neurotic Depression

Remember SAM F PIPE

S Sleep does not come easily

A Appetite is good

M Morning finds him feeling better

F Fatigued. No retardation

P Physical complaints common

I Insight present

P Projects. Personality good

E Evening finds him worse

Hebephrenic Schizophrenia

Remember DIM

D Dullness

I Irritability when interfered with
   Inconsistent behaviour
   Isolation

M Manneristic

Catatonic Schizophrenia

Excited Form
  Remember NAN

  N   Negativism—tendency to do the opposite of what others desire

  A   Anaesthetic skin

  N   Noisiness

Depressed Form
  Remember RMN

  R   Rigidity

  M   Mute

  N   Negativistic

Stuporous Form
  Remember FRMC

  F   Fixed postures

  R   Rigidity

  M   Mute

  C   Cyanosis of extremities

Paranoia

  Eccentrics: contrary individuals with peculiar fads
  Egocentrics: interested only in themselves
  Remember HEAR PQ

  H   Hypochondriacal

  E   Exalted

  A   Amorous

  R   Religious

  P   Persecutory

  Q   Querulant

Mania

Remember FEDOP

F	Flight of ideas
E	Elation
D	Delusions
O	Over-activity
P	Physical features

Melancholia (Psychotic or Endogenous Depression)

Remember DDDD

D	Dull
D	Depressed
D	Deluded
D	Death wishing

Delirious Mania

Remember AND TICH

A	Amnesic
N	Noisy
D	Delusions
T	Toxaemia
I	Insomnia
C	Confusion
H	Hallucinations

General Paralysis of the Insane

First Stage
  Remember FFFD

F	Flippant
F	Faulty in habits
F	Forgetful
D	Delusions of grandeur

Second Stage
  Remember FFF

F	Forty
F	Fatty
F	Fatuous

Third Stage
  Remember FFF

F	Fifty
F	Frisky
F	Fitty

Delirium Tremens

Remember HAD DT

H	Hallucinations (vivid; visual; they may see snakes and 'pink' elephants)
A	Apprehension
D	Dread
D	Disorientation
T	Tremor

Korsakow's Psychosis
Remember PATCH

P   Paramnesia (loss of memory with confabulation)

A   Acute delirium

T   Tender calves

C   Confabulation

H   Hallucinations (visual)

Pre-senile Dementia

1. ALZHEIMER'S DISEASE
Remember ACTS

A   Amnesia

C   Convulsions

T   Twitching, tremors

S   Spastic limbs; speech an incoherent gabble

2. PICK'S DISEASE
Remember DD

D   Deterioration mentally

D   Disintegration of language mechanism

3. HUNTINGTON'S CHOREA
Remember GCE S

G   Grimacing

C   Choreicform movements

E   Emotional

S   Speech explosive and grunting

Tabes Dorsalis
Remember PSP

P Pain—shooting

S Sensory disturbance; stamping gait

P Pupils—Argyll Robertson's. Accommodation reflex present, light reflex absent

Disseminated Sclerosis
Remember C RENT

C Clumsiness

R Reflexes exaggerated

E Euphoria

N Nystagmus (a constant fine jerky movement of the eyeballs)

T Tremor

Parkinsonism
Remember GERMS

G Gait—slow, shuffling, and running

E Expression mask-like; eyes stare unblinkingly

R Rigidity

M Movement—voluntary movement delayed; tremor

S Saliva—dribbling

SOME NOTABLE DIFFERENCES BETWEEN:—

Senile Dementia and	**Pre-senile Dementia**
Appears around age 60+	Appears at age 40+
Physical deterioration observable	Physical deterioration not observable
Mental deterioration gradual	Mental deterioration rapid
Fits not common	Fits common
Childishness marked	Childishness less marked
Muscle tone not unduly affected	Muscle tone increased

Anterograde Amnesia	**and**	**Retrograde Amnesia**

Anterograde Amnesia
Inability to fix impressions
Loss of memory confined to
  recent events
Causes
Undue self-absorption as in
  depression
Failure to attend
Confusion

and

Retrograde Amnesia
Inability to recall
Loss of memory confined
  to past events
Causes
Confusion
Mania
Injury to the brain, e.g.,
  post-concussional

Senile Paralysis Agitans

Dry skin
No dribbling of saliva
Tremor not marked
Lower jaw not dropped
Speech unintelligible
Posture not distorted

and

**Post-encephalitic
Paralysis Agitans**
Oily skin
Dribbling of saliva
Tremor marked
Lower jaw dropped
Speech intelligible
Posture distorted

Selected Features of Pre-senile Dementia

CONDITION	DOMINANT MENTAL FUNCTIONS AFFECTED	SIGNIFICANT PATHOLOGY
Alzheimer's disease	Memory	Brain atrophied. Convolutions narrowed. Sulci widen. Ventricles dilate. Degenerative patches or plaques are present
Pick's disease	Intelligence, thinking, and reasoning	Atrophy of both grey and white matter, especially in the frontal lobe. Degenerating cells are swollen. Atrophic changes appear as punched out areas—a sort of crater formation
Jakob-Creutzfeldt disease	Speech and motor activity, especially walking. Deterioration is rapid	Brain and spinal cord affected. Widespread deterioration

Selected Features of Pre-senile Dementia (*continued*)

CONDITION	DOMINANT MENTAL FUNCTIONS AFFECTED	SIGNIFICANT PATHOLOGY
Huntington's chorea	Motor activity— movements become unco-ordinated. Deterioration is gradual	Chronic meningitis and atrophy of the cerebellum

DOMINANT SYMPTOMS OBSERVABLE AMONG THE MENTALLY SICK

Disorders of Perception

Illusions; hallucinations (auditory hallucinations of noises such as buzzing, cracking, and ringing are called *acouasms*, whilst those of voices are referred to as *phonemes*).

Disorders of Consciousness

Clouding of consciousness; dream states; disorientation, unconsciousness.

Disorders of Memory

Amnesia (anterograde for recent events, retrograde for past events); faulty retention; lack of memory; excess of memory.

Disorders of Ideation

Flight of ideas
Circumstanciality
Distractability
Retardation
Poverty
Confusion
Neologisms
Obsession

Perseveration
Ruminations
Symbolic blocking
Knight's move
 (side-stepping)
Paramnesia (loss of
 memory with
 confabulation)

Approximate
 answers
 (a characteristic
 feature of Ganser
 syndrome, found
 in hysteria)
Morbid preoccu-
 pations

Disorders of Judgement

Delusions; lack of insight.

Disorders of Feeling

Exaltation	Ambivalence	Irritability
Euphoria	Lack of feeling	Fear
Elation	Apathy	Immaturity
Depression	Lability	Insecurity
Indifference	Anxiety	Over-expressiveness
	Aggression	

Disorders of Behaviour

Over-activity	Bland	Stereotype
Inhibition	Aversion (keeps	Ambitendency (half
Mannerisms	eyes turned away)	extends hand to
Tics	Adversion (keeps	examiner)
Tremors	eyes abnormally	Conversional
Akathesia (motor	fixed on the	(e.g., hysterical
restlessness)	examiner)	paralysis)

Disturbances of Will-power

Panic reactions	Stubbornness	Rigidity
Morbid suggestibility	⎧Echopraxia ⎨Echolalia ⎩Flexibilitas cereas⎫	Common in schizophrenia
Hesitation	Impulsiveness of	Compulsion
Impulsiveness of actions	speech	Over-assertiveness
	Deliberation and over-elaboration	Timidity

Disturbances of Conduct

Immodesty	Demonstrativeness	Suicidal
Exhibitionism	Over-modest	Righteous
Violence	Sexual deviations	Hoarding
Abuse	Isolation	Bullying and
Noisiness		threatening

Disturbances of Speech

Mutism	Echolalia	Word salad
Dysarthria	Slurred	Plausibility
Dysphasia	Staccato	Stutter
Aphasia	Monotonous,	Repetition
Perserveration	monosyllabic	Soliloquy (talking to
Verbigeration		oneself)

Disturbances of Sensations

Analgesia (lack of sensation)	Hyperaesthesia	Paraesthesia

Description of Appearance

EXPRESSION

Suspicious	Condescending	Anxious
Bland	Sullen	Excitable
Fatuous	Painful	Sulky
Expressionless	Appealing	Defiant
Dejected	Downcast	Self-conscious
Dull	Aggressive	Joyful

POSTURE

Bent	Drooping	Bizarre
Upright	shoulders	Casual
Elevated shoulders	Rigid or limp	Correct

DRESS

Casual	Inadequate	Creased
Showy	Dirty	Well-pressed
Unconventional	Clean	Quality of clothing
Conventional	Tidy	Consistency
	Untidy	

GUIDE TO THE RECEPTION AND ADMISSION OF PATIENTS TO HOSPITALS

Approach through the following headings.

Reception

1. Attitude of the nurse.
2. Facilities available.
3. Hospital image.

Admission

1. Routine and documentation.
2. Reception in the ward.
3. General duties of the nurse.

Reception

ATTITUDE OF THE NURSE

To be pleasant, uncritical, and interested in the patient as a person.

Pleasantness includes clean appearance, smartness of dress, and a smiling face.

She should conduct herself with poise and confidence.

FACILITIES AVAILABLE

A room where patient's visitors may be put at ease.

Books or periodicals during the period of waiting.

Someone to talk to.

Trolley or wheel-chair to be ready if required.

HOSPITAL IMAGE

A favourable image is useful to build morale and overcome insecurity.

A favourable image of the hospital may be created by showing real interest in the patient's comfort and welfare.

Get to know the patient's name beforehand so that he may be addressed by name. This is a friendly gesture.

Anticipate his wants, e.g., Does he want to go to the toilet? Might he be hungry?

Give the impression that you have been looking forward to meeting him.

Give the impression that you are efficient (capable) but kind.

Admission

ROUTINE AND DOCUMENTATION

Obtain statement of particulars. Name—correct spelling. Address. Name of own doctor. Religion. Age and sex. Telephone number if any. Name and address of nearest relative. Form of admission may vary; may be informal or formal. Check document to see if particulars are correct. Official record of admission is made.

RECEPTION INTO THE WARD

Introduce the patient to the ward. Show him round if that is possible.

Get through the preliminaries as soon as possible; check clothing and personal possessions.

Valuables to be checked by two people, and sent to the Nursing Office.

Patient may need a bath. Take height and weight afterwards. Inspect for bruises, etc., during bathing.

Report anything suspicious.

Patient to be prepared for examination by the doctor.

NURSES' DUTIES

1. To inform the doctor when patient is ready for examination.

2. To prepare the bed to receive the patient.

3. To observe the patient with the view of making a report on his general condition. Is he co-operative ? How does he look ? Are there any major symptoms to be seen. Does he look as if he is hearing voices ? Is he to be trusted ? How much observation do you think he will need ?

4. To help the patient to settle into the ward by (a) informing him of the routine and of what is expected of him, (b) planning and informing him of the routine for the first 24 hours at any rate.

5. To carry out doctor's instructions.

6. To keep the appropriate records and make the necessary report conscientiously.

Stay in hospital is not always the most pleasant of experiences, because patients have quite a lot of inconvenience to put up with. For one thing they have to accept dependency and a certain amount of unfavourable indignity associated with this, and as their movements and personal freedom are restricted it is not always easy to trust others. But this is what they are encouraged to do.

MATTERS AFFECTING PATIENTS

When a patient is admitted, it is essential to record what he brings in with him and to have a second person to check this. Informal patients especially are required to sign a receipt for personal property kept by them for their own use.

Patients are advised to bank any cash which they may have, and if they are not capable of doing this themselves the hospital should do it for them. Any money which accumulates by receiving pension and sickness benefits should also be put in the bank. Pocket-money for those who have no money of their own is paid to them weekly from an exchequer fund, and if they do some useful work within the hospital, even though this may be looked upon as part of their treatment, they should receive a little extra money as an encouragement.

During the first eight weeks in hospital the patient is entitled to receive his sickness benefit in full. After this, some reduction is made. Any patient who takes up work as part of his treatment is able to receive sickness benefit as well, as long as what he earns does not exceed a weekly sum determined by the Department of Health and Social Security.

Any mental patient not under the jurisdiction of the Court of Protection can make a valid will and any mental patient who is compulsorily detained in hospital can be a party to a contract.

The possessions of a patient who has died should be retained until instructions on how to dispose of them are received from the persons entitled to administer the estate of the deceased.

SELECTED LEGAL NOTES

1. The Hospital Management Committee is liable to compensate by way of damage anyone who is injured or suffers any loss through negligence of the hospital.

2. In the event of an injury or negligence, it is important to understand the routine for reporting such occurrences. Nothing should be put into writing unless reliable and truthful. Pain complained of by a patient should always be reported.

3. Drugs and equipment should always be checked and every possible step taken to prevent injury and neglect. This is absolutely essential.

4. In answering questions about a patient, refer the questioner to the person authorized to do this, unless of course you already hold this responsibility.

5. Poisons and dangerous drugs kept on the ward are the responsibility of the Ward Sister or Charge Nurse.

6. No person is allowed into a hospital unless he is invited, or is on official business following an official invitation to visit the hospital. Relatives visiting patients are excepted; doing this within the times laid down by the Hospital Management Committee is their prerogative.

Unauthorized persons would be classed as trespassers. This is one reason why a nurse, for example, is required to ask permission for bringing a friend into the hospital.

MENTAL HEALTH ACT, 1959

A new legislation which replaces the Lunacy Acts of 1890 and 1900, and Treatment Act, 1930.

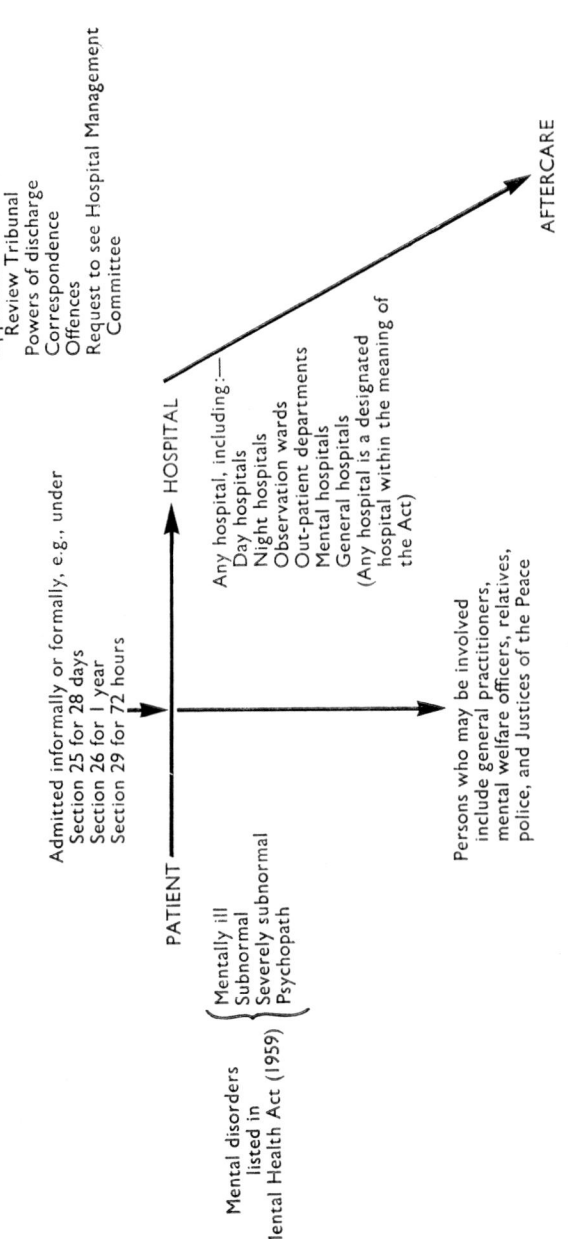

Fig. 4.—Plan of the hospital service for the mentally sick.

Sections of the Mental Health Act, 1959

SECTION

4. Definition and classification of mental disorders.
5. Informal admissions.
25. Admission for observation (28 days).
26. Admission for treatment (12 months).
29. Admission for observation in an emergency (3 days).
30. Application in respect of patient already in hospital.
36. Correspondence of patients.
39. Leave of absence.
47. Discharge of patients.
49. Definition of nearest relative.
60. Court Order.
71. Patient kept in custody during Her Majesty's pleasure.
122. Application to Mental Health Review Tribunal.
125–131. Offences.

135. Search for and removal of mentally disordered person by Mental Welfare Officer—Justice of the Peace directs.

136. Mentally disordered persons found in public places—removal.

THE MENTAL HEALTH REVIEW TRIBUNAL

Its constitution is considered at the end of the Act under the first schedule. It has legal, medical, and lay members.

Aims of This Act may be summarized as follows:—

1. To remove the stigma associated with certification of the mentally sick.

2. To make the admission of the mentally sick as informal as possible, and not to make it appear special and somewhat different from admissions of the physically sick.

3. To establish a unity of administration and supervision with the Ministry of Health.

4. Hospital care to be considered in the interest of the patient's health and safety.

5. To shift the care of the mentally sick from the hospital to the community.

6. Placing greater responsibility and duty on the nearest relative in respect of approving the application for admission, and appealing against the detention of the patient.

444

4444

444

Mental Disorders
Four types, as classified in this Act:—
1. Mental illness.
2. Severe subnormality.
3. Subnormality.
4. Psychopathy.

SEVERE SUBNORMALITY
Arrested or incomplete development of mind, with subnormality of intelligence, of such a nature or degree that the patient is incapable of living an independent life, or guarding himself against serious exploitation.

SUBNORMALITY
Arrested or incomplete development of mind not amounting to severe subnormality, but including subnormality of intelligence, of such a nature or degree which requires or is susceptible to medical treatment, or other special care or training of patient.

PSYCHOPATHIC DISORDER
Persistent disorder or disability of mind (with or without subnormality of intelligence), resulting in abnormally aggressive or seriously irresponsible conduct, and which requires or is susceptible to medical treatment.

Functions of the Local Health Authority in Connexion with This Act are to:—
1. Supply and maintain residential accommodation for the mentally sick not removed to hospital.
2. Carry out periodical inspection of residents.
3. Care for persons in residence, e.g., those kept for observation.
4. Provide centres or other facilities for the training or occupation of patients, e.g., those in guardianship.
5. Appoint officers to act as Mental Health Officers.
6. Approve of practitioner for making medical recommendation for the detention of patients.
7. Allow for payment to cover personal expenses of those under the age of 16 years in residential accommodation.
8. Accept application for guardianship on behalf of any other person, and consequently to approve guardianship.

Duties of the Mental Welfare Officer (M.W.O.)
1. To make application for the admission of a patient into hospital or for guardianship.

2. May enter or inspect premises (not being a hospital) in the area of that authority in which a mentally disordered patient is living, if the patient is not under proper care.

3. May apply to County Court for the Court to make appointment for a person to act as nearest relative.

Patients may either be admitted into hospital or placed under guardianship, whichever is the more suitable for the patient.

Admission of a Patient

May be admitted informally or compulsorily.

INFORMAL ADMISSION

As simple as any procedure can be. The procedure here is similar for all kinds of patients.

COMPULSORY ADMISSION

This may be for (a) observation or (b) treatment.

For observation, without being an emergency (Section 25):—
For a period of 28 days.
Two medical recommendations are required.
Application to be made within 14 days of seeing the patient.
Medical recommendations may be made together or at an interval of not more than 7 days, and this before the application is made.
Patient to be admitted within a 14-day period after submitting the application.

For observation in an emergency (Section 29):—
Patient may be taken to a hospital any time within a period of 3 days beginning with the date on which the patient was examined by the doctor giving the medical recommendation.
Patient is detained for 3 days.
Only *one* medical recommendation is sufficient for this period.

For treatment (Section 26):—
Admission for a period of 1 year in the first instance, repeated for another year if necessary, then renewed every 2 years.
Two medical recommendations are required.
Application to be made within a period of 14 days of seeing the patient.
Medical recommendations may be made together, or at an interval of not more than 7 days, and this before the application is made.

Patient to be admitted within the 14-day period from the date of submitting the application.

Patient to be medically examined within a period of 2 months before the period of hospital detention ceases. This is for the purpose of making further application if necessary.

An informal patient already admitted for 3 days may be detained under Section 30.

Safeguards against Wrongful Detention

1. The two medical recommendations.

2. Patient and/or relative may appeal to a Mental Health Tribunal within a period of 6 months following the admission of the patient.

Nearest relative may call in own doctor to examine the patient in private for the purpose of making application to the Review Tribunal.

3. The doctor in charge of the patient has the power to discharge the patient.

4. The Hospital Management Committee has the power to discharge the patient.

5. Nearest relative may order his discharge.

Restriction on Discharge by Nearest Relative

1. Nearest relative must give 72 hours' notice for the purpose of discharging the patient.

2. Responsible medical officer (doctor in charge of the patient) may furnish medical evidence, and submit same to the Hospital Management Committee for the purpose of barring the order of discharge made by the nearest relative. This medical evidence is made only when it is considered that the patient if discharged would be likely to act in a manner dangerous to other persons or to himself.

No further order for the discharge of the patient may be made by the nearest relative for a period of 6 months.

Relative may, within a period of 28 days of being informed of this, apply to a Mental Health Review Tribunal of the patient.

Discharge of a Patient

PATIENT RECEIVED FOR OBSERVATION

By the doctor in charge of the patient, or by the Hospital Management Committee.

PATIENT RECEIVED FOR TREATMENT
By the doctor in charge of the patient.
By the Hospital Management Committee.
By the nearest relative of the patient.

PATIENT RECEIVED ON A COURT ORDER (ADMISSION FOR TREATMENT)
By the doctor in charge of the patient.
By the Hospital Management Committee.
Patient discharged to the Court, or to a place named by the Court.
Secretary of State may discharge a patient any time.
Nearest relative of patient so detained may apply to Mental Health Review Tribunal within the period of 12 months, and in any subsequent period of 12 months.
Patient may apply within a period of 6 months.
Admission of patients from a Court is made on an order based on 2 medical recommendations given orally in evidence at the hearing. The court may decide to authorize admission to hospital, or place patients under guardianship of the Local Health Authority.
A Juvenile Court cannot make such an order, unless the parent of the juvenile understands what is involved.

Guardianship

Application to be made within a period of 14 days to the Local Authority, and beginning with the date the patient was last examined by M.O. before giving recommendation. Procedure for making application is similar as for the admission of patient to hospital for treatment.

Correspondence of Patients

Correspondence of patients received into hospital for observation or for treatment, may be sent to the following:—
The Minister of Health.
Any M.P.
The Master or Deputy Master or any other officer of the Court of Protection (this being a section of the High Court).
The Hospital Management Committee.
Any person having the power to discharge the patient.
The Mental Health Review Tribunal, any time during the period when a patient is allowed to apply.

Any postal packet addressed to a patient in hospital may be withheld from them only at the discretion of the doctor in charge of the patient.

'Nearest Relative' means Any of the Following:—

   i. Husband or wife.
   ii. Son or daughter.
   iii. Father.
   iv. Mother.
   v. Brother or sister.
   vi. Grandparent.
   vii. Grandchild.
   viii. Uncle or aunt.
   ix. Nephew or niece.

Leave of Absence for Patients received for Treatment

This may be made indefinitely, or may be periodically renewed without the patient being in hospital.

Absence without Leave of Patients admitted for Treatment

May not be returned if 28 days or more have elapsed (6 months in the case of a psychopath or a subnormal patient).

QUESTIONS ON THE MENTAL HEALTH ACT, 1959

1. What is meant by a designated hospital within the meaning of the Act?
2. Is Section 5 a declaration (yes or no).
3. Does the Board of Control exist?
4. Does the Mental Health Act describe a voluntary status?
5. Is it possible to abuse Section 29?
6. If so, how?
7. Within what period following a ban on the discharge of a patient may the nearest relative apply to the Mental Health Tribunal?
8. What is the composition of the Mental Health Review Tribunal?
9. What is the Court of Protection?
10. What does it do?
11. What is the function of the Public Receiver in respect of the mentally ill?
12. Is forgery an offence within the Act?

13. What has been described in the Act as a 'disorder or disability of mind'?
14. Who authorizes a patient to be removed from his home into hospital against his will?
15. Where may a patient be detained at Her Majesty's pleasure?
16. Give an example of a special hospital.
17. Can admission to a psychiatric hospital be a condition of a probation order (yes or no)?
18. Is the word 'psychiatry' used in the Mental Health Act (yes or no)?
19. What is the use of Section 30 other than to detain an informal patient?
20. Does the Act state that a responsible Medical Officer is allowed to open the letters of patients detained on Section 26 (yes or no)?
21. What does Section 4 of the Mental Health Act refer to?
22. Do you find any information about the Samaritans in the Mental Health Act?
23. Can children be admitted for treatment under Section 26 of the Mental Health Act (yes or no)?
24. Has a responsible medical officer the authority to open a letter addressed to a patient admitted for observation (yes or no)?
25. How many Mental Health Review Tribunals are there nationally. 1, 2, 5, 10, or more than 10?

(*Answers on p.* 147)

DEFINITION QUIZZES

Read the definitions carefully one at a time, and from the list of words on the right, choose the one which you consider fits the particular definition. Insert the letter by which the word is identified in the bracket at the side of the appropriate definition.

QUIZ I

1. Abnormal rage which sometimes occurs following an epileptic fit.   ( )
2. A misinterpretation of a sensory impression.   ( )
3. Loss of memory, or impaired memory. ( )
4. Anxiety associated with an anticipated event or experience.   ( )

5. A readiness to reject or accept, or to act in a predetermined way. ( )
6. A violent crippling emotion. ( )   *A.* Apprehension.
7. A strong or intense emotion of a short   *B.* Post-traumatic.
   duration. ( )   *C.* Attitude.
8. Susceptibility to emotional stimula-   *D.* Furor.
   tion. ( )   *E.* Passion.
9. Imitation of movements. ( )   *F.* Echopraxia.
10. Loss of voice. ( )   *G.* Confabulation.
11. Waxwork-like posture maintained for   *H.* Illusion.
   long periods. ( )   *I.* Aphonia.
12. New words coined by a patient. ( )   *J.* Therapeutic.
13. Recurrent mood-swings of elation   *K.* Neologisms.
   and depression. ( )   *L.* Temperament.
14. An emotion prevailing over a vary-   *M.* Mood.
   ing period of time. ( )   *N.* Dissociation.
15. Splitting up of consciousness by   *O.* Flexibilitas
   ideas forced into it from the un-   cereas.
   conscious. ( )   *P.* Rumination.
16. Constant repetitive recollection of   *Q.* Dysphasia.
   past experiences. ( )   *R.* Cyclothymia.
17. Speech which is difficult, indistinct,   *S.* Verbigeration.
   and unintelligible. ( )   *T.* Sentiment.
18. An emotional attitude composed of a   *U.* Projection.
   cluster of emotions. ( )   *V.* Tremor.
19. Continuous purposeless repetition of   *W.* Status
   words and phrases. ( )   epilepticus.
20. To attach such sentiments as love or   *X.* Transference.
   hate to a substitute, or to direct a   *Y.* Amnesia.
   sentiment to something or someone   *Z.* Fear.
   other than the original. ( )
21. A mechanism by which personal faults, weaknesses, etc., are attributed to other people and to things outside ourselves. ( )
22. Trembling, shaking. ( )
23. A condition in which a series of epileptic fits occur in succession. ( )
24. Following injury. ( )
25. Relating to treatment. ( )

QUIZ II

1. Tingling sensations. ( )
2. The time of life at which the sexual organs become active. ( )
3. Refusal to co-operate and doing the opposite of that asked. ( )
4. To believe that nothing exists or that everything is dead. A form of delusion. ( )
5. Arising from mental causes rather than from physical ones. ( )
6. The process by which a re-pressed emotional trauma is con-verted into a physical symptom. ( )
7. A condition without known cause. ( )
8. To derive pleasure from inflicting pain. ( )
9. Sleep walking. ( )
10. A condition in which there is an uncontrollable desire for sleep. ( )
11. A fear of our own nervousness. ( )
12. A fixed obsessive fear. ( )
13. Mental subnormality present from birth or from an early age. ( )
14. A rapid shift from one idea to another in conversation. ( )
15. State of bewilderment associated with muddled thought. ( )
16. Returning to an infantile level of behaviour. ( )
17. The process of directing repressed impulses into socially acceptable channels. ( )
18. Inability to state the time or place, or to identify oneself correctly. ( )
19. A false belief which is impervious to reasoning. ( )
20. The process by which painful experiences are pushed into the unconscious. ( )

A. Psychogenic.
B. Somnambulism.
C. Sadistic.
D. Narcolepsy.
E. Anxiety.
F. Phobia.
G. Confusion.
H. Paraesthesia.
I. Repression.
J. Sublimation.
K. Puberty.
L. Regression.
M. Conversion.
N. Disorientation.
O. Displacement.
P. Negativism.
Q. Hypnosis.
R. Nihilistic.
S. Reaction formation.
T. Delusion.
U. Idiopathic.
V. Astasia.
W. Hypochondriasis.
X. Amentia.
Y. Rationalization.
Z. Flight of ideas.

21. An apparently plausible excuse to justify an unconventional act. ( )
22. Taking one's feelings out on some harmless object. ( )
23. Reacting to a situation with an attitude which is the opposite to that in the unconscious. ( )
24. Sleep-like state induced by suggestion. ( )
25. Excessive preoccupation with health and functions of the body. ( )

(*Answers on p.* 148)

MISCELLANY
DID YOU KNOW THAT ... ?

The World Health Organization has now recommended that the terms 'drug addiction' and 'habituation' be replaced by the single one of *drug dependence*.

Indian hemp or cannabis is a plant which grows in most parts of the world. The resin (hashish) or the dried flowers or leaf (marijuana) may be smoked, and the elixir may be drunk, whilst marijuana can also be eaten or taken in the form of snuff.

The Dangerous Drugs Act, 1967, makes it:—

1. Obligatory for general practitioners to notify cases of addiction to drugs controlled under the Act to the Chief Medical Officer of the Drug Branch of the Home Office.

2. Unlawful to prescribe heroin or cocaine to an addict except when this is done by doctors specially licensed to do so.

The object of this Act is to exert some control on drugs which had been over-prescribed.

Principles of management of drug dependence may be considered under these headings:—

1. *Prevention* through education, control, and supervision.

2. *Treatment and routine management* in a hospital or a special centre. And apart from routine care and relatively strict supervision treatment may involve either one or a combination of the following: aversion therapy, modified insulin, continuous narcosis, psychotherapy (individual and group), treating the underlying cause, use of tranquillizers to control behaviour, special attention to physical health.

3. *Rehabilitation*.

It is never possible for a man to misuse his reason except deliberately. This is the basis of the legal view of mental illness, incorporated in the *M'Naghten Rule*, formulated in 1843.

These days it is usual when describing personality to assess both physique and temperament in the manner described by Dr. William Sheldon:—

Physique	*Temperament*
Ectomorphic (thin)	Cerebrotonic (self-conscious and
Endomorphic (fat)	emotionally inhibited)

Signs of Drug Dependence

DRUG	FACE	PULSE	SLEEP	BEHAVIOUR*
Amphetamines (pep pills), e.g., dexedrine or black bombers, drinamyl or French blues	Flushed. Dry mouth. Chewing or teeth grinding movements. Pupils dilated	Fast	Wants none	Intolerant, argumentative, aggressive, and over-confident. Mood swings—euphoria to depression. Poor appetite
Barbiturates (sleepers)	Pale. Tired eyes. Pupils dilated	May be fast or slow	Feels drowsy	Clumsy. Unsteady walk. Appears drunk. Uninhibited
L.S.D. (Lysergic-diethylamide)	May look excited or vacant. Pupils dilated	Fast	Wants none	Excitement common. Infantile behaviour. Euphoria. Mood changes. Some may have a wonderful feeling of well-being
Cannabis (Indian hemp; 'pot')	Pupils dilated. Flushed. Blood-shot eyes. Dry mouth	Fast	Wants none	Appears drunk. Laughs for no reason. Mood changes. Some may become over-anxious and fearful
Heroin. A derivative of morphine. Referred to as the hard drug, because of the difficulty in breaking the dependency. Sudden withdrawal of the drug produces severe distress and extreme restlessness. Convulsions may also occur. The patient may even collapse and die suddenly	Eyes sensitive to bright light. Pupils pin-point	Fast	Drowsy and yawns	Slow slurred speech. Elation followed by anxiety and agitation. Personal neglect and social irresponsibility. Hand tremor

* Overall behaviour is unpredictable and depends in many ways on the person's basic disposition.

Mesomorphic (muscular)   Viscerotonic (sociable and lover of
comfort)
Somatotonic (assertive and
aggressive)

Personality may be a combination of any two—one type of physique with one type of temperament.

Of the number of emotionally disturbed patients seen at out-patients throughout the country:—

50 per cent suffer from anxiety.

25 per cent suffer from neurotic depression.

20 per cent suffer from hysteria and overlapping conditions.

3 per cent suffer from phobias.

1 per cent suffer from anorexia nervosa, neurasthenia, tics, and occupational cramps.

Between 30 and 35 per cent of the population show *preclinical neurosis syndrome*. Its roots are deep in the physical and emotional background of the individual.

The main symptoms of preclinical neurosis are insomnia, depression, attack of nerves, and undue irritability.

One-third of the population is born with or develops nervous systems which are more prone to neurotic illness than the remaining two-thirds.

There is a hard core of neurotic patients who are ill most or all of the time. These are constitutionally anxious and worried and form about 5 per cent of the population.

Sympathy and kindness and pleasant physical surroundings increase overt neurosis.

A functional disturbance is often due to emotional disturbance within either the family or the person's intimate group, and this prevents them from getting on well with each other. One affects the other adversely, so to speak.

Treating the disturbance involves diagnosing the pattern of emotional forces within the group and attempting to readjust it. Doing this is therapeutic and is often termed *Vector therapy*.

One person locked in an intense emotional relationship with another, like a mother with a child, and who conveys two conflicting signals to the other continuously, may bind the second person with perplexity, suspicion, doubt, and unresponsiveness, through not being able to decide on what to do. This has been referred to as the *double bind* and is conceived as a possible cause of schizophrenia. It must be most disturbing especially for a child to be caught in a permanent dilemma of not knowing whether mother loves him or not.

According to Bleuler, schizophrenia contains both primary and secondary symptoms.

Primary symptoms are splits, so to speak.

Affect splits away from thought.

The train of thought splits and gives rise to muddled thinking. There is an inability to keep the mind focused on any one thing. Attention is directed to many different things at the same time.

Ideas of reference—thinking that people are talking about him, and the world of make-believe which he creates—are evidence of a split in his sense of reality.

Secondary symptoms follow as defences and may take the form of over-activity and excitement or of mute inactivity and withdrawal into himself. This is usually referred to as *autism*. Both are attempts to deny the fact that reality is slipping away from him.

Paranoid symptoms may appear as the ego disintegrates and fails to keep unconscious impulses in check. And in an attempt to free itself of these disturbing impulses, the mind projects them to the outside world. Thoughts and feelings from the unconscious are projected outwards but come back again to form hallucinations and delusions.

Most authorities recognize *childhood autism* as a condition characterized by emotional detachment from people, unusual movements and postures, extreme sensitivity to stimuli, intolerance of change, and language difficulties. It occurs more commonly in boys than girls. The cause is unknown and is not easily treated.

The tendency nowadays is to call paranoid schizophrenia in late middle age or in the elderly, *paraphrenia*. Paraphrenia has had a number of meanings. Once it was used as an alternative for paranoid or as a diagnostic intermediate between paranoia and paranoid schizophrenia. It was also taken as an inclusive term for paranoia and schizophrenia.

Depression which results from a disturbance in the mother/child relationship is called *anaclinic depression*.

In practice one way of deciding on whether or not a patient is anxious, agitated, or latently aggressive is by watching the hands.

With *anxiety*, there is often a restrained-controlled hand restlessness. There is a sort of 'doing and undoing' type of hand movement, e.g., rolling a handkerchief up and then unrolling and smoothing it out before rolling it up again, and so on.

With *agitation* there is a 'picking' type of hand restlessness. They may pick at clothing, at the skin, at the nails, and so forth. Also, there is often restlessness of both hands and feet.

Where there is *latent aggression* a 'finger-tapping' type of restlessness is common. The person is also more impulsively restless.

Nail-biting, apart from being a disorder of habit, is probably one of the commonest types of restless activity associated with anxiety, mild agitation, and latent aggression at one and the same time.

The type of hand restlessness which may be associated with self-consciousness is the holding with feeling or touching type. Hands seek things for holding and for allowing the fingers to move restlessly over and around them.

Alcoholism is a disease and to the alcoholic it is a frightening and baffling experience. As a drug of addiction, alcohol produces symptoms similar to those associated with other drugs of addiction. There is craving, increased tolerance, and withdrawal symptoms when alcohol is suddenly withdrawn. The main withdrawal symptoms are those of shock, restlessness, and excitement. The average alcoholic is by nature fearful, anxious, and tense. He has also a tendency to self-justifications; his family and society are wrong, never himself, and as time goes on he becomes a plausible liar. The usual treatment is one of aversion, followed by a period of rehabilitation.

Alcoholics Anonymous help a good deal, for they will visit patients in hospital and provide help and encouragement when the patient is ready for discharge. A number of homosexuals are often alcoholic, and the drinking homosexual is practically incurable.

The Samaritans are dedicated groups of people trained to help those who contemplate or have unsuccessfully attempted suicide. In one way they could be looked upon as 'Suicides Anonymous'.

Many *epileptics* are dependent, somewhat childish, selfish, easily slighted, anxious to enlist the sympathy of others whilst lacking in sympathy themselves. The self-righteousness which they display is reflected in their frequent religious preoccupation.

Epileptics are prone to fits and many become irritable, restless, and difficult to manage before having a fit. By the use of anti-convulsants such as epanutin and phenobarbitone, however, most are able to live a relatively normal life.

Fits may be of two forms:—
a. Grand mal (a major convulsion).
b. Petit mal (a fleeting loss of consciousness for a few seconds).

A major convulsion, after passing through the aura, cry, tonic, and clonic stages, ends in sleep, whilst a petit mal may lead to automatism, a state in which the patient acts in a strange way. Some may become restless and violent, whilst others just wander about aimlessly. A violent rage which may follow a fit is called a furor, whilst an amnesic wandering episode is called a fugue.

ELECTRO-ENCEPHALOGRAPHY (E.E.G)

Electro-encephalogram: a record.
Electro-encephalograph: the apparatus.
Electro-encephalography: the procedure.

This is a highly specialized technique by which the electrical activity of the brain can be recorded.

There are four frequencies:—
The fast: Beta
The intermediate: Alpha and theta
The slow: Delta

In children the records fluctuate between theta and alpha rhythm until about the age of 11 years.

Absence of alpha rhythm in adults is normally a sign of vivid visual imagination.

Alpha rhythm scans for pattern.

Theta rhythm scans for pleasure.

(In bad-tempered adults, especially in those with an unusual tendency to aggressive behaviour, the theta rhythm is often prominent and may swing through quite a large area of the brain.)

The alpha rhythms, prominent when the eyes are shut and the mind is at rest, disappear whenever the eyes are opened and when a subject makes a mental effort—for example, while doing a sum in mental arithmetic.

People can be classified into three types according to the absence or presence of alpha rhythms. A group with persistent activity is known as the *P type*, while the larger group whose alpha rhythms are responsive is known as the *R type*. A third group has no significant alpha rhythms and is known as the *M type*.

When one considers the different 'characters' of the three personality groups, P, R, and M, and the effect of their different ways of thinking, it is little wonder that we do not see the same things in the same way. Next time you argue with your friends, think of this.

Normal rhythm in the average adult when awake:—

Regular alpha rhythm blocked on opening the eyes.
Beta activity may occur in frontal and central regions.
Theta activity disappears after the age of 25 years.

Sleep record

Reduction in alpha activity.
Bilateral theta rhythms appear instead.
As sleep deepens, delta rhythm becomes prominent.

Abnormal record

Spike-and-wave complexes—three cycles per second associated with petit mal.
Rhythmic spikes with intervening slow waves common in grand mal.
Square flat tops to the waves may signify masked epilepsy.
Delta activity in the waking state may be associated with cerebral tumour.

Prior to an E.E.G.

All drugs should be continued, including regular anti-epileptic medication, except Librium and Valium, which should be stopped for 1 week.
An E.E.G. should not be done for 1 week after lumbar puncture, or for 6 weeks after E.C.T.
Hair grease and lacquer may interfere with recording.
Administration of barbiturates abolishes superficial activity of the brain, but reveals deep activity.

TRAINING OF NURSES ON THE WARDS

On joining a ward or a department, trainee nurses are expected to hand their ward schedules to the nurse in charge. Schedules are records of all the practical experiences which a nurse in training acquires. It is hoped that the nurse in charge will keep the schedules in a place where they can be seen and where they are accessible. Otherwise they are easily forgotten and lost. Schedules should be checked and adjusted at least once weekly.

Following each lecture block, a list of the procedures which the tutor considers could be practised at ward level could be inserted just inside the front cover of each schedule. This, it is hoped, would serve as a guide for the nurse in charge to appreciate the immediate practical needs of the nurse concerned and of the stage of training reached.

It is also hoped that Ward Sisters/Charge Nurses will, at least once a week, be able to set aside a definite period for meeting trainee nurses informally, individually or preferably as a group, to discuss problems of mutual interest as they affect the ward, the training of the nurse, and staff–patient relationships.

Here are some suggestions on how to meet the educational needs of trainee nurses on the wards. I am sure that you are aware of many of these already.

1. On entry to the ward, make sure that the nurse is presented with a basic plan of her duties and that she is informed of what is expected of her.

2. Realize that all nurses in training are highly suggestible and will copy incorrect techniques (bad habits) more easily than correct ones (good habits).

3. Do not take for granted that the nurse knows what she has been asked to do. Find out if she does know first. If she doesn't, then arrange for her to be instructed. Never leave in ignorance.

4. Build on what the nurse knows rather than on what she does not know, and whenever possible say 'do' rather than 'don't'.

5. Ensure that whatever is being done conforms with the standard of etiquette and ethics particular to the profession.

6. Avoid asking difficult questions and giving complicated explanations.

7. Try not to baffle the nurses with science and technical jargon.

8. Avoid that pet hobby-horse, that favourite subject which we personally may enjoy talking about, but which may prove boring or confusing to others.

9. Set projects and ask the nurse to report back.

10. Encourage nurses to do things with patients rather than by themselves. A nurse should be made to realize that her place is with patients.

11. Attempt, whenever possible, to inform the nurse about what you yourself may be doing.

12. Encourage patient-centred and group-centred assignments. Delegate trainee nurses to look after a patient or a group of patients. Give them the scope and responsibilities to plan and to organize activities and to care for the patients in their own way, but naturally under discreet supervision.

13. Make sure that nurses in training are brought into group discussions and staff meetings and are allowed to accompany the doctors on their ward rounds.

14. From time to time check to find out if the nurse knows as much as she should about the patients.

15. When necessary, assist the nurse to compile nursing studies of particular patients. Guide on the choice of patients for this purpose.

16. From time to time select a patient and demonstrate the nursing needs peculiar to that patient.

17. Whenever possible, attach a first-year nurse to a more senior nurse, so that the more experienced nurse will serve as mentor, guide, and confidante during the first few months of training.

18. Trainee nurses in psychiatry should learn more about inter-personal relationships than about trays and trolleys.

19. Encourage nurses to ask questions and to challenge—but within reason, of course—time-honoured customs, techniques, and procedures.

20. Ask for their opinions, advice, and suggestions.

21. Acquire the habit of asking why. Why do you do that ? Why should it be like this ? etc. The four leading questions which the nurse in charge should be asking are:—

Does the nurse know what she is doing ?

Does she know how to do it ?

Does she know why she is doing it ?

Is she aware of the dangers ?

22. Avoid talking for more than ten minutes at a time without getting the nurses' participation in what is being discussed.

23. Avoid cutting corners, but be as realistic and practical as possible in the way procedures are performed.

24. Encourage the nurse to become methodical in the way that she performs her job. This, of course, is learnt as much by example as it is by instruction.

25. Encourage nurses working in clinical areas to keep procedure charts.

It is also hoped that Ward Sisters/Charge Nurses, Clinical Instructors (when available), and Tutors will continue to work closely together with mutual respect and appreciation of the valuable contribution which each makes not only to the training of nurses, but also to the care of patients and to the morale of the hospital as a whole.

We live as we learn and learn as we live.

A PLAN FOR WRITING A STUDY OF A PSYCHIATRIC PATIENT (A CASE NOTE)

This is to be developed in three stages:—

1. Ask the ward sister if she can give you a brief account of the patient's background and if possible the diagnosis.

2. Read your textbook, and find out what it says there about this condition.

3. Carry out discreet observations yourself.

You are not allowed to consult the patient's case note unless permitted by the consultant psychiatrist in charge of the patient.

Write the case note away from the ward.

Do not put the patient's name anywhere.

Skill rests with you finding out as much as you can about the patient yourself.

Writing the Case Note

1. GIVE A GENERAL ACCOUNT

Give a general picture of the patient as a person.

Bring in his background; any special problems which have dominated the patient's life.

Has he got a family ? Has he travelled much ?

Has he made a successful career for himself, etc. ?

What is your general impression of the patient as a person ?

Has he a pleasant personality ?

Is he temperamental ?

Is he forceful or not in his relationships with others ?

What contribution does he make to the ward ?

Is he helpful on the ward ?

Is he sociable ?

How often does he speak and what does he talk about ?

Has he any special likes or dislikes, etc. ?

2. Consider Him as a Patient

First, write down a concise summary of this particular condition—the diagnosis—as described in the textbook.

Next, record methodically your own observations.

Write about the patient's appearance, expressions, standard of cleanliness, the way he stands.

Next consider:—

a. Behaviour

What of his toilet, eating, and sleeping habits?

Are the habits conventional and regular or not?

How does he conduct himself? Is he modest? Is he conventional?

Does he show respect or is he disrespectful and unruly, etc.?

Is he a worker or an idler?

b. Peculiarities

Mannerisms and compulsive actions, if any.

c. Special features

Describe what you observe. Avoid assuming too much.

Is there evidence of hallucinations, delusions, illusions, confusion?

Is there over-activity or under-activity, aggression and violence?

Are there any signs of exhibitionism?

Is he impulsive, restless, garrulous, argumentative, noisy, etc.?

Also observe and record what is said and note the tone of voice, the type of words used, the frequency and volume of what is said.

What were you able to do for this patient, in an attempt to promote comfort, well-being, and pleasantness?

Report on supervision, accepting that this involves care and management. Through care we satisfy needs and protect, whilst as we manage we control and direct behaviour.

How did you manipulate difficult behaviour, if any?

How much persuasion was used?

What kind of suggestion is the most suitable for this type of patient?

Could you control behaviour by the use of incentives?

What is the routine for the patient? What special demands did this make on you?

Were the patient's psychological needs satisfied?

Did you have to change the environment in any way to suit the patient?

Have you been of any assistance to the psychiatrist?

What observation of yours did the psychiatrist consider a useful contribution ?

What special treatment is the patient on ? Did you help in any way ?

This of course is a mere guide. The quality of a case study depends a good deal upon the interest, imagination, and conscientiousness of the observer.

PLAN OF A PSYCHIATRIC NURSING REPORT

1. *Appearance*
   a. Expression (bland, happy, miserable, suspicious, aggressive, etc.).
   b. Posture (upright, bent, stooping, etc.).
   c. Physique (fat, thin, tall, short, etc.).
   d. Dress (tidy, untidy, smart, indifferent, etc.).
   e. Cleanliness (always, often, sometimes, never, etc.).
2. *Attitude to the situation* (hostile, friendly, anxious, distrustful, etc.).
3. *Behaviour*
   a. General activity (quiet, restless, impulsive, etc.).
   b. Conduct (reaction to, and relationship with, others).
      i. Co-operation in respect of nursing care.
      ii. Co-operation in respect of treatment.
      iii. Interests.
      iv. Needs.
      v. Dependency.
   c. Habits (toilet, sleep, exercise, eating, occupation, etc.; whether acceptable, could be improved, or unacceptable).
4. *Conversation* (what is said, how it is said, how often).
5. *Disposition* (intolerant, insecure, mature, immature).
6. *Any other observations.*

A MISCELLANY OF ORAL QUESTIONS MANY OF WHICH COULD BE USED AS A BASIS FOR DISCUSSION

What do you find annoying about neurotic patients ?

How does a neurotic patient differ from a normal person ?

What is anxiety ? How do you distinguish between anxiety and apprehension ?

What is meant by the word demonstrative ?

What effect does fear have on the body ?
Which hormone is released into the blood-stream when fear is
    experienced ?

Some people consider that an attitude to a situation is often more
    important than the situation itself. Would you agree ?
Would you accept that basically every patient wants to be friendly ?
What are the main features of immaturity ?
How would you handle immature patients ?
How does the body respond to pleasure ?

Would you consider diarrhoea to be dirty ?
How would you remove faeces from the floor of a dormitory ?
Which terms are preferred to the following:—

Asylum	Escape	Superior
Mental deficiency	Certification	Voluntary
Wet and dirty	Refractory	Cruelty
Chronic	Custodial	Neglect

How would you check on the bowel habits of a neurotic patient ?
A patient comes up to you and states 'I have not had my bowels
    open yet. Could I have an aperient ?' What would you give
    him ? What is the composition of faeces ?

Which type of patient is most likely to spend a great deal of time in
    the toilet ?
Give examples of compulsive behaviour.
What are the special problems associated with nursing obsessional
    patients ?
What is the meaning of the word paranoid ?
How do you *manage* patients ? What does the word management
    involve ?
What effect has emotional tension on the body ?

Are hysterical patients generally inhibited or excitable ?
What does a person who panics lose ?
How would you deal with a patient who panics ?
What is anaphylaxis ? Could penicillin give rise to anaphylaxis ?
    How could it be avoided ? What is the immediate treatment for
    anaphylaxis ? Which substance released in the body is
    responsible for this ?

How would you assess the efficiency of a junior nurse ?
How much responsibility should a first-year nurse be allowed ?
Would you permit a first-year student nurse to give injections ?
What is the difference between sterilization and disinfection ?
What are the functions of the skin ?
What effect does stimulation of the vagus nerve have on the body ?

A patient at home is placed on Section 26. Who authorizes his
    removal to hospital against his wishes ?
Can a nurse refuse to carry out doctor's instructions ?
Of what importance are ethics to a nurse ?
What do you consider are good manners ?
What effect does exercise have on the body ?
If a person had a lot of cheek, would you accept that he had a
    great deal of initiative ? What is initiative ?

What are the symptoms of hypoglycaemia ? What may produce
    hypoglycaemia ?
What is the value of modified insulin therapy ? Give an account of
    how this is carried out.
Is insulin a hormone or an enzyme ? Which organ secretes
    insulin ? What other functions does this organ have ?

What treatments are used in psychiatry ?
What is psychotherapy ?
Can you as a nurse perform psychotherapy ?
Explain how you would persuade a patient to stay in the ward
    instead of going to the Occupational Therapy Department.

What bacteria are usually found on the human skin ?
What bacteria would you expect to find in the dust of a geriatric
    ward ?
How much cleanliness do you think is necessary on such a ward ?

Which part of the ward merits the most attention ?
What is the meaning of the word geriatric ?
What advantages are there in growing old ?
What is a reflex action ?

Should a nurse assess the personality of a patient ? How would
    you set about doing this ?

What would be your impression of the relationship between a nurse and a patient if you were to read this kind of report: 'Mrs. J. Jackson lifted a chair and deliberately smashed a window in the day room.'

What do you consider are the general characteristics of adolescents ?

Some people consider that adolescence is a normal fleeting psychopathic phase in a person's life. Would you agree ?

What is intelligence ? Can this be measured ? How is it assessed ? Name one test used.

What special consideration would a patient with superior intelligence and education require ?

What are the functions of a child guidance clinic ?

What effect does recreation have on the body ?

Who employs a Mental Welfare Officer ?

What are the duties of a Mental Welfare Officer ?

What are the principles of nursing hysterical patients ?

What is meant when it is said that hysterical patients exaggerate reactions ?

A patient may be said to have recovered volition. What is volition ?

What effect does a delusion of persecution have on the body ?

How would you reassure a patient who was vomiting profusely ?

What complications may be associated with severe, continuous vomiting ? Could this be due to fear ?

How would you know if a patient was frightened ?

What are the functions of the sympathetic branch of the nervous system ?

What are peripheral nerves ?

What do you know about the Mental Health Review Tribunal ?

If I wanted information about the constitution of the Mental Health Review Tribunal, where would I look ?

In what ways are mentally sick people protected whilst in hospital ?

Explain how you would admit a new patient who was very distressed at the time of admission ?

How might the relatives behave ?

Could they project their anxieties in any way ? Explain how you would realize that this was being done.

Should a nurse learn about psychopathology ?

What help would you give a patient who, after being detained in hospital for three months, wishes to be discharged against medical advice ?

What help would you give a patient who complains that a student nurse has revealed knowledge of personal details which had been disclosed only to the doctor ?

What do you know about the human mind ?

What effect does sleep have on the body ?

What is a habit ?

How would you distinguish between behaviour and conduct ?

What is meant by motivation ?

Give some idea of how an inactive long-stay patient may be remotivated.

What would you consider are the qualities of a psychiatric nurse ?

Is there such a thing as an ideal psychiatric nurse ?

What effect does a hot bath have on the body ?

What action does the liver have on fat ?

What do you consider is meant by psychiatric first aid ?

What may produce an emotional shock ?

How may a person react to an emotional shock ?

Is it necessary for psychiatric nurses to undergo a special three-year course of training ? Why ?

What is the meaning of the word hygiene ?

What is mental hygiene ?

What effect would lack of cleanliness have on the body ?

If you were in charge of a ward, how would you attempt to promote a good staff relationship ?

What do you consider are the qualities of a leader ?

What are your views about pupil-nurse training ?

What would you do if you saw a junior nurse hitting a patient ?

How would you deal with a patient who was classed as a bully ?

How would you make milk more digestible for a physically ill patient ?

What effect would starvation have on the body ?

In what ways can a patient be encouraged to express his individuality ?

Would you look suspiciously at an elderly patient who is giving a younger patient much attention and protection ? What could be the reasons for this ?

What is meant by the word transference ? Could a nurse make use of this in her nursing relationships ?

A patient is transferred from one ward to another. What special problems of adjustment may occur ?

What effect does aggression have on the body ?

Name some common emotions.

What is abreaction ? What does it involve ? Of what value is this ?

What form of occupation would you consider suitable for a hypomanic patient ?

What are the aims of occupational therapy ?

Is it necessary to have this organized ?

How would you assess progress ?

What are the uses of water in the body ?

How much water is there in the body ?

How would you organize a group of patients for a discussion ?

What is the value of discussions ? Are there any disadvantages to having discussions ?

What types of fractures do you know of ?

What first aid would you administer to a patient with a fractured femur ?

What is the composition of bone ? What movements occur at the hip-joint ?

What effect would a long stay in bed have on the body ?

What is meant by the word 'tact' ? When would you use tact ?

What is meant by rehabilitation ? What methods are in general use.

What are the duties of a nurse in the event of a patient absenting himself without leave ?

Which vitamins contribute to the health of the skin ?

What is the treatment for scabies ?

What effect would toxaemia have on the body ?

Why is it necessary for a psychiatric nurse to have a good character ?

It has been said that the most useful tool which a psychiatric nurse possesses is her own personality. Would you agree ?

What first-aid treatment would you give a patient who some few minutes before swallowed a lethal dose of aspirin ?

What effect would aspirin have on the body ?

Is the statement 'once a suicide, always a suicide' true from your experience ?

You are asked to tell an apprehensive patient that the visitors he was expecting are now unable to come. How would you do this ?

What precautions are taken on your ward to prevent accidents ?

What would you observe about an unconscious patient ? Of what value are these observations ?

How may patients behave if they are insecure ?

How would you help such patients ?

Often it is not what a patient says that is important, but what he does not say. Would you agree ?

What effect does emotional tension have on the body ?

What is insight ?

Many patients ask for drugs as a way of achieving extra nursing contact. Would you agree ?

What should a nurse guard against when trying to find out the mental state of a new patient ?

What would you do if a patient woke up in the middle of the night with a severe attack of asthma ?

In what illness do you expect to find conversional symptoms ?

How would you manage a patient who has a functional paralysis of both legs ? Would behaviour therapy be of any value here ?

What effect would poor circulation of blood have on the body ?

What do you consider are the main differences between psychopathy and a hysterical personality ?

Psychiatric patients, it has been suggested, may benefit from being grouped on admission according to their social status. What do you think ?

To whom may a patient admitted for treatment send sealed letters ?

It has been suggested that introverted people should be discouraged from taking up psychiatric nursing. Why is this ?

What effect would fatigue have on the body ?

How would you prevent fatigue ?

What factors in the ward environment may tend to make a patient aggressive ?

How would you deal with a patient who is threatening other patients ?

How could you help a junior nurse who is afraid of an aggressive patient ?

What is meant by the term 'special hospitals' as used in the Mental Health Act, 1959.

Which organization is responsible for administering the hospital service in England and Wales.

What are the functions of bile ?

What psychological reactions may a physically handicapped patient experience ?

How much privacy should a psychiatric patient have ?

What could you do to make sure that a patient gets the privacy he needs ?

It has been suggested that if a patient refuses to get up, out of bed, he should be left where he is. What do you think ?

How much discipline do you consider necessary for an admission ward ? What is discipline ?

What do you know about a therapeutic community ? What are the disadvantages of such a community ?

What effect does inactivity have on the body ?

How does voluntary muscle obtain its energy for contraction ?

When you breathe in, does the diaphragm rise or fall ?

EXAMPLES OF PROJECTS SUITABLE FOR STUDENT NURSES

1. Choose two wards.
2. Find out what the sitting position of each patient is. Is there a regular pattern ?
3. What are the reasons for this ?
4. Has any attempt ever been made to change these positions ?
5. What is the general pattern of the sitting positions now in being ?

1. What books do patients read ?
2. Which is the most popular type ?
3. How much reading is done and how long for ?
4. How are books, etc., issued to the ward ?

5. How many books are available and is the number issued adequate ?

1. Select two or three patients.
2. Find out how much and how far patients move in the course of, say, two hours.
3. What is the purpose and reason for this movement ?
4. What is the pattern of movement ? Is it repetitive or not ?
5. Should it be changed ?

1. Select a ward.
2. Find out how many patients have visitors and how many do not.
3. Are those who have visitors concerned about it ?
4. When visitors arrive, do those patients who do not usually have any move out of the ward ? What do they do ?
5. Is there any need for compensation here ?

1. Select a ward.
2. How many of the patients on this ward do you consider as asocial ?
3. What are the reasons for this ?
4. Should they be allowed to remain asocial or not ?
5. Seek the view of the ward staff on this point.

1. Select a ward.
2. Look out for examples of mental mechanisms.
3. Which is the most prominent ?
4. What are the reasons for this ?
5. Are the nurses on the ward aware of the mechanisms which you consider exist ?

1. Select a ward.
2. What is the average weight of the patients ?
3. Are they overweight ?
4. Do they over-eat ?
5. How much choice of food is there on the ward ?

1. Select a ward.
2. How many dominant independent patients are there on the ward ?

3. Also, how many dependent patients are there ?
4. Is there any evidence of bullying among the patients ?
5. How many patients are status conscious ?

1. Select a ward.
2. How would you assess boredom on this ward ?
3. How many patients talk to themselves ?
4. Do they have their hands in their pockets as they talk ?
5. How many patients have their hands in their pockets ?

1. Select a ward.
2. Find out if there is a common topic of conversation among a group of patients.
3. Do they form groups by themselves ?
4. What are the reasons for this ?
5. Should it be encouraged or discouraged ? What are your views ?

1. Is there a common interest which the patients share ?
2. If there is, how do you account for this ?
3. Of what advantage or disadvantage is this ?
4. How do you cultivate a common interest among a group of patients ?

1. How many patients with special skills or abilities are there on the ward ?
2. How much use is made of these ?
3. What are the factors influencing their use or disuse ?
4. How are they fostered ?

1. Select a ward.
2. Do patients use nick-names ?
3. How have these come about ?
4. Have they any value ?

1. Select a ward.
2. What are the general personal and social standards of the average patient ?
3. Are those reflective of what the average person has outside the hospital ?
4. How sociable is the average patient ?

1. Select a ward.
2. How many deluded and hallucinated patients are there on this ward?
3. What forms do these delusions and hallucinations take?
4. Do they give rise to any problems? If so, what?

1. Select six patients.
2. Compare their background from their case notes. (Get permission first, of course.)
3. Would you say that their background has had any influence on their personality and on their illness?
4. How much do their varying backgrounds contribute to their being different as persons?
5. How much do they remember about their backgrounds?

AID TO ANSWERING EXAMINATION QUESTIONS

1. If a question involves care, management, or nursing of a patient, then consider:—

I	Inspection
A	Anticipation, Activity Affection, Achievement
C	Checking Communication
R	Recording, Reporting, Reassurance Routine, Responsibility
O	Observation
I	Inter-personal relationships

2. If a question asks for the causes of a social problem, consider:—

i. Frustration.
ii. Low morale.
iii. Failure to satisfy needs.
iv. Fear and anxiety.
v. Jealousy and rivalry.
vi. Temperament—impulsive, aggressive.
vii. Attitude.
viii. Delusions and hallucinations if it refers to the mentally sick.

3. If a question asks for aims or purpose, consider:—
Protection.
Prevention.
Promotion.
And to answer how to protect, prevent, and promote, consider:—
Hospitalization, assessment, diagnosis, treatment, care, and rehabilitation (training, recreation, resocialization). Aftercare with financial aid.

4. If a question asks for the value, advantages, or disadvantages, consider the following aspects:—
   i. Hygiene.
  ii. Health.
 iii. Aesthetic.
 iv. Economic.
  v. Educational.
 vi. Moral.
 vii. Social.
viii. Practical.

5. If a question is the essay type, *plan* it.
Consider:—
Introduction (brief).
Body
   i.
  ii. } Main ideas.
 iii.
Conclusion (brief).
Write about 35 lines in 30 minutes.
When a question is asked as 'discuss', consider for and against what has been stated.

6. If a question is concerned with the care of a physically ill patient, then consider:—
   i. Bed: position, linen.
  ii. Comfort.
 iii. Morale.
 iv. Nursing technique.
  v. Prevention of complications.
 vi. Ventilation, heating, and lighting.
 vii. Diet, fluids.

viii. Bowels.

ix. Cleanliness.

x. Records and recording.

General Note

Try to be methodical—start at the beginning and work through your reasoning step by step.

Try to picture a situation in your mind.

Whenever possible try to recall similar circumstances from your experience.

Watch spelling.

Write full sentences whenever possible.

Draw a simple diagram if you think it would help to illustrate your answers.

DATES OF OUTSTANDING EVENTS IN THE HISTORY OF PSYCHIATRY

2500 –500 B.C.	Behaviour disturbances were regarded as evidence of possession by evil spirits.
500 B.C. –200 A.D.	Graeco-Roman Rationalism—The Pythagorean school recognized the brain as the organ of intellectual activity and mental illness as evidence of its disorders.
490 A.D.	First Mental Hospital founded in Jerusalem.
800–1500	The Middle Ages. A period dominated by the persecution of the insane as witches and demons. The principal authority for the entire persecution of the insane was a book called *The Witches' Hammer* written by two monks.
1736	Laws against witchcraft were cancelled or repealed in the United Kingdom.
1743	An Act for the chaining of dangerous lunatics was passed.
1765	King George III was afflicted with mental illness.
1792	William Tuke, a Quaker, and a cocoa and tea merchant, founded the Retreat Hospital at York for the treatment of insane persons without restraint.
1798	Philippe Pinel removed the chains that restrained the insane patients of the Bicêtre Hospital in Paris.
1808	Justices in Quarter Sessions were empowered to set up County Asylums.
1820	King George III died mad, deaf, and blind.

1840   Dorothea Lynda Dix, a retired American school-
        teacher, campaigned for improvement of conditions
        in mental hospitals.

1843   Nursing lectures were given at Surrey Asylum.

1845   The first Lunacy Act. It made it obligatory for
        Quarter Sessions to take care of paupers of un-
        sound mind.

1854   A proper training scheme for nurses was arranged at
        Crighton Institute, Dumfries.

1856   John Conolly, Medical Superintendent of Hanwell
        Asylum, gave up his professorship at University
        College, London, when all his efforts to introduce
        psychiatry into the teaching curriculum were
        obstructed.

1885   The so-called 'Red Handbook', a textbook for mental
        nurses, was produced.

1888   Local Government Act placed the responsibility for
        the care of the mentally unsound upon the local
        authorities.

1890   The first lasting Act of Parliament was passed to direct
        the care of persons of unsound mind.

1891   The first examination for mental nurses was held by
        the Royal Medico-Psychological Association.

1893   Psycho-analytic movement was started by Sigmund
        Freud.

1896   Kraeplin, a German, differentiated three major groups
        of mental illness—dementia praecox, manic depres-
        sive psychosis, and paranoia.

1903   Binet, a Frenchman, experimented with intelligence
        testing.

1907   Major symptoms of hysteria described by Janet.

1911   The term 'schizophrenia' was coined by Bleuler, a
        German.

1915   Jung introduced analytical psychology.

1916   Adler propounded his views on individual psychology.

1920   Prolonged narcosis used by Klaesi.

1924   First human electro-encephalograph by Berger.

1930   Mental Treatment Rules were introduced to supple-
        ment the 1890 Act. These established the voluntary
        status of out-patients' clinics.

1934   Insulin coma therapy introduced by Sakel.

1936	Convulsion therapy introduced by von Meduna.
1936	Prefrontal leucotomy introduced by Moniz.
1939	Electro-convulsive therapy introduced by Cerletti and Bini.
1939	Sigmund Freud died.
1948	The General Nursing Council took over the training of psychiatric nurses.
1954	The age of the tranquillizers began.
1957	A drastic revision of the syllabus for the training of psychiatric nurses occurred.
1959	A new Mental Health Act was introduced to replace the 1890 Act. This did away with the certification of patients.
1960	Gradual decrease in the number of patients resident in mental hospitals.
	Of the number of patients being admitted, a large percentage was now psycho-geriatric. There were more women than men in this category.
	The need for beds for mental illness was recognized as being 1·8 beds per 1000 of the population.
1971	Today, psychiatry and psychiatric nursing are respected professions.

ANSWERS TO QUESTIONS ON THE MENTAL HEALTH ACT, 1959 (pp. 117-18)

1. Any hospital—general, psychiatric, subnormal, etc.
2. Yes.
3. No.
4. No.
5. Yes.
6. By admitting a patient and holding him for three days merely for the convenience of relatives.
7. 28 days.
8. Lay, medical, and legal.
9. Office of the Supreme Court.
10. Managing and administering patient's property and affairs.
11. Acts within the area of residence of the patient on behalf of the Court of Protection, and manages and administers patient's property and affairs whilst the patient is mentally incapacitated and until the Judge who appointed him as receiver terminates the appointment.
12. Yes.
13. Psychopathy.
14. Justice of the Peace—a Magistrate.
15. In a special hospital.
16. Broadmoor and Rampton.
17. Yes.

18. No.
19. To allow:—
     a. For the doctor in charge of the patient to furnish the Hospital Management Committee with a report in writing on why he considers the patient should be admitted to hospital.
     b. For the Management Committee to deliberate on what action to take.
20. No, except in exceptional circumstances (*see* Section 36, subsection 3, of the Act).
21. Definition and classification of mental disorders.
22. No.
23. Yes.
24. No, except in exceptional circumstances (*see* Section 36, subsection 3, of the Act).
25. More than 10.

ANSWERS TO DEFINITION QUIZZES (pp. 118-121)

Quiz I	*Quiz II*
1. *D.*	1. *H.*
2. *H.*	2. *K.*
3. *Y.*	3. *P.*
4. *A.*	4. *R.*
5. *C.*	5. *A.*
6. *Z.*	6. *M.*
7. *E.*	7. *U.*
8. *L.*	8. *C.*
9. *F.*	9. *B.*
10. *I.*	10. *D.*
11. *O.*	11. *E.*
12. *K.*	12. *F.*
13. *R.*	13. *X.*
14. *M.*	14. *Z.*
15. *N.*	15. *G.*
16. *P.*	16. *L.*
17. *Q.*	17. *J.*
18. *T.*	18. *N.*
19. *S.*	19. *T.*
20. *X.*	20. *I.*
21. *U.*	21. *Y.*
22. *V.*	22. *O.*
23. *W.*	23. *S.*
24. *B.*	24. *Q.*
25. *J.*	25. *W.*

SECTION III
MEDICAL

INTRODUCTION

MOST of us would do almost anything to remain healthy and active, for we know that without health and the ability to move about freely, there is little chance of living a successful, happy, and prosperous life. Illness begets fear, fear distress, and betwixt the two there is much anguish and discomfort. And whilst most of us dread illness, a few are lucky in that they are able to accept illness philosophically with confidence.

For the majority, the mere thought of coming to hospital is alarming; it is a frightening and a bewildering experience. So, in an attempt to minimize the insecurity and anxiety associated with illness and hospitalization we either blame ourselves or others for our indisposition.

Those of us who blame ourselves tend to become irritable, moody, depressed, sullen, and apathetic, whilst those who blame others may become hostile, aggressive, haughty, defiant, suspicious, over-talkative, or restless. Awkward and difficult behaviour, or so it may appear to a nurse, invariably arises from anxiety and insecurity associated with being ill and with being in a strange environment.

A nurse learns to accept awkwardness as a sign of insecurity, and goes out of her way to make the patient comfortable and happy. A nurse gives much of herself, in the knowledge that, if a patient is to feel secure and is to have confidence in the nursing and medical staff, it is imperative that she gives of her best. And, of course, this is what most nurses do with tact, compassion, and kindness.

The overall duties of a nurse when caring for a physically ill patient are to:—

Attend to the patient's needs.

Carry out doctor's instructions.

Maintain a standard of ethical conduct, favourable to the well-being of the patients.

Make accurate observations and report these.

Be interested in patients as people.

PHYSICAL ILL HEALTH

The causes of physical ill health may be considered under the following headings, using the mnemonic PIGDOT.

Psychological in that emotional upsets disturb body functions and give rise to signs and symptoms of ill health. (A sign is that which is visible, e.g., a bruise; a symptom is that which is experienced and which cannot be seen, but which the patient complains of.)

Infection due to the presence of bacteria.

Growths.

Deficiency and degeneration. Deficiency, of oxygen, of blood, or of nutrients, and so on. Degeneration, of a structure; usually this is a progressive irreversible process.

Obstruction either to the flow of air, blood, or intestinal content, and so on.

Trauma (injury) to any part of the body.

The signs and symptoms of physical illness vary with the cause, and many of the more common conditions are caused by infections. As an aid to learning, it may be of value to group signs and symptoms as those due to:—

    i. Disturbance of function.

    ii. Irritation.

    iii. Congestion, obstruction, and compression.

    iv. Toxaemia—the presence of bacterial poison in the blood.

EXAMPLE

Pneumonia: inflammation of the lungs. Their normal function is to draw air in, to allow O_2 to enter the blood, and to allow CO_2 to pass out of the blood into the lungs.

Interference with these functions gives rise to two dominant 'signs', dyspnoea or difficult breathing, and cyanosis due to an increase in the amount of 'free' haemoglobin in the blood—haemoglobin with no oxygen attached to it. (Retention of CO_2 in the blood increases its acidity and, if uncorrected, would give rise to 'symptoms' of acidosis.)

The inflammation itself would be a source of discomfort, of possible pain, and of irritation. Coughing would be due to the irritation. And whilst this may be dry at first, it soon becomes moist as the secretion of mucus is increased. Coughing finally results in the expectoration of sputum. (Sputum is infected mucus and may vary in thickness, stickiness, and colour.) It is described as mucoid if it only consists of mucus, purulent if it has more pus than mucus, and muco-purulent if it is a mixture of the two.

Congestion, which for general purposes may be viewed as a swelling, may obstruct the free flow of air to and from the lungs.

Toxaemia, a condition associated with the presence of bacterial poison in the blood, may, as the blood circulates through the various systems of the body, disturb the normal activities of these systems, and give rise to a collection of symptoms, commonly referred to as 'constitutional symptoms'. These include fever, tachycardia (a fast pulse), rapid breathing, loss of appetite, nausea, vomiting, constipation, headache, a restless sleep, general tiredness, and the passage of small quantities of highly concentrated and highly coloured urine.

Mental symptoms may also appear, and they vary in degree according to the severity of the toxaemia. Irritability with restlessness and insomnia are the symptoms most commonly seen.

When the toxaemia is extreme, restlessness becomes more marked, and there is confusion with illusions, hallucinations, and delusions. In this state the patient is said to be delirious. Voices are often abusive, and may provoke the patient to acts of violence or to suicidal attempts. Conversation becomes incoherent, and the patient is completely unable to give relevant answers to questions. He mutters and rambles on incessantly.

Please note that the convention nowadays is to use the term 'symptoms' loosely for both signs and symptoms. Apart from a few exceptions, 'constitutional symptoms', as those listed above, are standard to most physical illnesses caused by an infection. With this knowledge, and an understanding of human biology, it is possible to build up the signs and symptoms of other infective illnesses for ourselves.

The treatments available may be described as:—

a. *General* when it just involves rest and routine nursing care.

b. *Symptomatic*.

c. *Specific*: to treat the cause of the illness, and to build the body's resistance to the infection. The body itself attempts to do this by increasing the number of white blood-cells in the blood-stream. An increase in the white blood-cell population is called *leucocytosis*.

Infection

An invasion by pathogenic bacteria which may be local or general. A localized limited reaction to infection is called *inflammation*.

A more generalized reaction would produce a fever, and most possibly a *rigor*. A rigor has three phases to it—a cold phase with shivering, a hot phase, and a sweaty one. Rigors are very exhausting, and require a good deal of nursing care.

Allergy

Hypersensitivity of body-cells to one or more specific proteins, e.g., hay fever and urticaria.

Anaphylaxis

A sudden severe allergic reaction accompanied by shock and possible collapse.

The symptoms are due to the histamine which is released in the body. Adrenaline must be administered immediately to counteract this.

Pathogenic (Disease-producing) Bacteria

Visible only under a microscope.

For simplicity and convenience, these may be grouped as follows:—

1. COCCI (coccus for one).

A coccus can be a ball-, egg-, or bean-shaped organism.

Any number of these may be grouped together in various ways, and may exist in clusters, in pairs, or in the form of a chain. A cluster of cocci is known as a *staphylococcus*, a pair as a *diplococcus*, and a chain as a *streptococcus*.

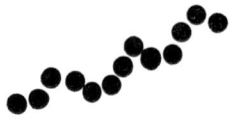

A streptococcus   A staphylococcus

Streptococci are usually found in the mouth, nose, and throat of normal people.

One likely place where staphylococci may be found is the skin.

There are many varieties, and one of the most powerful is the *haemolytic*. This variety produces a highly dangerous poison or toxin which may damage the heart muscle and valves. It is this variety which is invariably the cause of a severe sore throat with a very rapid pulse. Whilst a sore throat may be due to other causes, it is the rapid pulse accompanying it which suggests a streptococcal infection.

Illnesses caused by one variety or another of streptococci are:—

Sore throat; scarlet fever (sore throat with a rash as it is called today); erysipelas; rheumatic fever; nephritis (inflammation of the kidneys); pneumonia.

If streptococci are contained in a boil or an abscess, they produce a thin, watery, blood-stained pus.

There are two main varieties. *Albus* which produces a white coloured pus, and *Aureus* which produces a yellow pus. Both varieties are found in boils, abscesses, and carbuncles.

Staphylococci and the toxin which they produce can give rise to symptoms of gastro-enteritis. This is one reason why it is important to wash our hands before handling food.

Staphylococci off unwashed hands and from contaminated food may give rise to sickness and diarrhoea, or to what may often be classed as a form of food poisoning.

A germ which produces pus is usually described as a *pyogenes*.

Sulphonamides, penicillin, and tetracyclines are the drugs chosen for the treatment of a coccal infection. Unfortunately, however, some cocci may after a time become resistant to them.

Bean-shaped cocci which may be found singly or in pairs are referred to as *neisseria*.

2. ROD-SHAPED BACTERIA (BACILLI)

A bacillus   —spore

Some of these are capable of producing a protective envelope or a capsule called a *spore* which develops usually at the end of the rod. When its surroundings are unfavourable, it draws itself into this envelope or shell, and remains there until conditions improve.

A spore cannot be destroyed by boiling, a much higher temperature is needed. Steam under pressure is one method often used for this purpose.

Examples of rod-shaped bacteria:—

Haemophilus: very small rods causing influenza and whooping cough.

Salmonella: small rods, responsible for typhoid, paratyphoid, and a variety of gastro-enteritis.

Shigella: small rods, of which *Proteus* is a variety. This organism is sometimes associated with urinary infection.

Spirochaetae: slender rods twisted like a 'corkscrew'; one variety of spirochaetae causes syphilis.

Clostridia: rods with spores. They cause tetanus (lock-jaw) and gas gangrene.

Corynebacteria: thick-skinned rods responsible for diphtheria, often club-shaped, hence the prefix *coryne*.

Both the clostridia and the corynebacteria produce a powerful toxin which damages nerves and causes paralysis.

Mycobacteria: slender rods, a variety of which is the cause of pulmonary tuberculosis.

Pseudomonae: of which the organism pyocyaneus, which produces green-coloured pus, is one example.

3. VIRUSES

These are smaller than the general run of bacteria, and can only be seen by the aid of an electron microscope.

They are highly specific in action.

They do not grow in ordinary food material (culture media) used for growing bacteria in the laboratory. Many, however, seem to grow well in the tissues of the developing chick embryo.

The following diseases are caused by viruses:—

Chicken pox.

Smallpox.

Mumps.

Poliomyelitis.

Measles.

German measles.

Common cold.

Influenza.

ISOLATION

Consider:—
1. Selection and preparation of a suitable room or area.
2. Duties of the nurse, to herself, to the patient, and to the community.

Selection and Preparation of a Room

Room to be quiet, accessible, convenient, easily ventilated, heated, lighted, and cleaned.

Furniture to be kept down to a minimum. No mats or carpets.

Necessary equipment—crockery, change of linen, receptacles for used linen, bed-pan, and urinal—to be kept within the area and clearly marked.

Duties of the Nurse to Herself

To have frequent breaks, adequate rest, sleep, exercise, recreation, and plenty of good food.

To report if not feeling well.

To maintain a high standard of personal cleanliness.

Duties to the Patient

To give full nursing care conscientiously.

To maintain comfort and morale.

Duties to the Community

To take all necessary steps to avoid carrying the infection and to educate and train the less informed in the precautions to be taken.

To maintain a satisfactory level of supervision at all times.

DISINFECTION

Bedclothes

Bed linen and personal linen are to be laundered and disinfected daily.

Washing for 10 minutes at 65° F. (17° C.) in an alkaline soap solution containing 0·5 per cent sodium metasilicate.

Alternative, but less efficient

Soak in general disinfectant, e.g., Sudol 1 in 80 for 12 hours.

Soiled Linen

Use disposable polythene bags, sewn on one side with alginate thread.

In the laundry these bags are immersed in water at a temperature of 50° C. containing soda 1 per cent. The thread dissolves, liberating the contents of the bag. This content is held in this solution at a temperature of 50° C. for 20 minutes and then boiled for 10 minutes.

Alternative, but less efficient
Soak in general disinfectant, e.g., Sudol 1 in 80 for 12 hours.

Blankets

Soiled: low temperature washing with suitable detergent, e.g., quarternary ammonium compound.

Unsoiled: either autoclave with formaldehyde or ethylene oxide, or subject to steam at sub-atmospheric pressure.

Rooms

Fumigate with formaldehyde (electrically heating 500 ml. of formalin with 1000 ml. of water).

Room is sealed.

Fumigation is done overnight. Two days airing of room afterwards.

Alternative
Use B.P.L. (B. Propiolactone) vapour.

Spray 500 ml. per 1000 cu. ft. of sealed room.

A relative humidity of 70 per cent is necessary.

Fabrics are removed, drawers are opened.

Fan distributes the vapours.

Two-hour exposure is enough and the room can be re-occupied in 10–18 hours if well ventilated.

CLEANING

Rooms

Mop with hot water and detergent.

Furniture

Damp clean daily, using either Chloros 10 per cent, chlorhexidine 0·1 per cent, cetrimide 0·1 per cent, or 70 per cent alcohol.

Baths and Wash Basins

Rinse with 0·1 per cent hypochloride solution with a detergent in hot water.

Bed-pans and Urinals

Steam sterilize.

Brushes

Store in 0·02 per cent aqueous chlorhexidine solution.
Before use immerse for 1 minute in 0·5 per cent alcoholic chlorhexidine.

Clinical Thermometers

Either store in 0·2 per cent chlorhexidine, 2 per cent gluteraldehyde, or in 70 per cent alcohol.

Excreta (Faeces and Urine)

Use general disinfectant 1 in 10 white disinfectant such as Izal for 2 hours.
For general purposes and for non-surgical equipment and crockery, Izal or Sudol are recommended.

A BRIEF ACCOUNT OF THE MAIN MEDICAL CONDITIONS WHICH A PSYCHIATRIC NURSE MAY ENCOUNTER

OSTEO-ARTHRITIS

Occurs in late middle life and is due to chronic degenerative changes in the large joints of the body such as the hips and knees.
The joints creak.
Pain is variable, ranging from a dull boring sensation to a severe sharp one.
Movement becomes difficult.
After some months of suffering, the muscles controlling the affected joints begin to waste.
The skin over the joints becomes tight, glistening, and white.

Treatment

GENERAL
Reassurance.
Reduction of body-weight if this is excessive.
Rest when the pain is severe.
SYMPTOMATIC
Relief of pain by the aid of a hot-water bottle or a hot application, e.g., Kaolin poultice.

The use of drugs to relieve pain, to reduce inflammation, and to increase mobility. Such drugs include aspirin, indocid, butazolidin.

SPECIFIC

None known.

Surgery may be resorted to, either to fix the joint or to reshape it.

RHEUMATOID ARTHRITIS

This is said to be commoner in females than males, and may occur at any age from childhood to old age. It is a chronic inflammatory and degenerative condition occurring in the smaller joints, such as the fingers and toes.

To start with, there is malaise, fever, and swelling of joints. The joints which are painful seem worse at night.

Movement of the affected joints becomes difficult.

Muscles controlling the joints soon waste with disuse, and as the joints become deformed.

After some time, as anaemia appears, the patient begins to feel generally unwell.

The cause is unknown.

As the condition progresses it cripples.

Treatment

GENERAL

Bed-rest with full nursing care in the early stages, and whilst the acute phase lasts.

SYMPTOMATIC

Analgesics, e.g., salicylates, to reduce pain.

Physiotherapy, massage, and electrical treatment.

SPECIFIC

Gold injections.

Drugs: Corticotrophin.
Prednisolone.
Betamethasone.
Triamcinolone.

TONSILLITIS

Inflammation of the tonsils and the fauces (the area which surrounds them).

The commonest organisms which cause tonsillitis are the common cold virus and the streptococci.

Signs and symptoms vary with the organism and the degree of toxaemia present. Constitutional symptoms are common.

The throat is naturally sore and there is some difficulty in swallowing.

The lymphatic glands in the neck, especially the ones behind the angles of the jaw, become enlarged and tender.

Spots of pus may be visible on the surface of the tonsil.

Treatment

GENERAL

The patient should remain in bed in a comfortable, warm room until the temperature has fallen to normal. A light diet consisting of jellies, milk foods, ice cream, sweetened fruit juice, is satisfactory.

SYMPTOMATIC AND PALLIATIVE

Gargles and lozenges.

SPECIFIC

Sulphonamide and penicillin.

BRONCHITIS (ACUTE)

Acute catarrhal inflammation of the bronchi.

May occur at any age.

Symptoms are those of cold, with cough, pain in chest, especially behind the lower end of the sternum.

The chest may be wheezy and there is a good deal of sputum.

Treatment

GENERAL

Nurse in a warm room in a fairly upright position.

Give plenty of hot drinks.

SYMPTOMATIC

Inhalation of steam medicated with tincture of benzoin compound if the chest is tight and painful and if there is a dry cough.

A bronchitis kettle may be used for a few hours or inhalations of a detergent mist, e.g., Alevaire.

Linctus, e.g., codeine, to suppress cough.

A light kaolin poultice to the front of the chest may be found soothing.

Sedatives may be necessary if insomnia is severe.

Tonics of iron with cod-liver oil or vitamin-A concentrate may help to improve the general condition.

SPECIFIC

Sulphonamides and penicillin.

Tetracyclines are used only on occasions.

CHRONIC BRONCHITIS

A chronic catarrhal inflammation of the bronchi.

Occurs in middle and old age and is more common in men than women.

Cough is very troublesome at night and there is shortness of breath.

There is much sputum and much wheezing.

A certain amount of apprehension and anxiety may develop especially at night. Some patients may even become irritable and argumentative.

Treatment

GENERAL

A dry equable climate.

Should spend as much time as possible out of doors in mild weather.

Deep breathing is encouraged.

Tobacco and alcohol to be forbidden.

Stout patients should reduce weight because obesity increases dyspnoea.

SYMPTOMATIC

Postural drainage to drain the sputum.

Expectorants, e.g., ammonia and ipecacuanha mixture B.P.C. (B.P.C. means British Pharmaceutical Codex).

Suppress cough at night with a linctus.

Antispasmodics such as stramonium compound mixture B.P.C. may be given if there is bronchial spasm.

SPECIFIC

None known.

Antibiotics merely help during the winter months to prevent and combat lung infection.

PNEUMONIA

May occur at any age.

There are two main varieties—lobar, when one or more lobes of the lungs are inflamed, and broncho-, when there are scattered areas of inflammation in both lungs.

Constitutional symptoms are prominent and to start with there may be a rigor (a cold shivering attack).

The face is anxious and flushed with a degree of cyanosis.

There is pain in the side affected.

The sputum is rusty due to the presence of minute streaks of blood.

Temperature rises to about 101–103° F. (38–40° C. approx.).

Lips may be covered with herpes.

Some patients become confused and restless.

Treatment

GENERAL

Full nursing care in a warm, well ventilated room.

Diet to be liquid or semi-solid in the early stages. Fruit drinks sweetened with sugar or syrup, fruit jellies, milk, soups, bread, butter, and weak tea are all acceptable.

Keep in bed and do not allow up until after 7 days' freedom from fever.

SYMPTOMATIC

Kaolin poultice to painful side.

Sedatives if restless.

Digoxin if there is cardiac weakness, and hydrocortisone if there is circulatory failure.

Oxygen therapy.

SPECIFIC

Sulphonamides and penicillin.

Streptomycin is of value in some pneumonias.

Tetracyclines and chloramphenicol have no advantages over the older remedies.

PLEURISY

Inflammation of the pleura; usually secondary to pneumonia.

Other than some constitutional symptoms there is usually a severe sharp pain in the side affected.

There may be some coughing with slight dyspnoea.

Dyspnoea may be marked if there is effusion (collection of fluid in the pleural cavity) as well.

Treatment

GENERAL

Rest in bed and a light diet with plenty of fluids.

SYMPTOMATIC

Kaolin poultice for the chest pain.

A linctus to suppress the cough.

Pleural effusions may have to be drained.

Breathing exercise as the condition improves.

SPECIFIC

Varies with the cause.

When there is no known cause, about 30 per cent of the patients concerned develop pulmonary tuberculosis later.

Antibiotics may be of use if the organism causing the condition is known.

PULMONARY TUBERCULOSIS

Acute pulmonary tuberculosis is a tuberculous pneumonia, running a rapid course.

Symptoms are constitutional with a cough, dyspnoea, and a high fever.

Profuse sweating occurs, especially at night.

There is a rapid loss of weight and wasting.

Chronic pulmonary tuberculosis is a tuberculous infection of the lungs.

Symptoms are constitutional with fever at night.

Sputum may be blood-stained.

The cheeks are flushed.

The patient sweats profusely at night.

There is clubbing of the fingers.

Anaemia occurs.

Depression and suicidal tendencies may appear.

Diagnostic Tests

X-ray.

Estimation of blood sedimentation rate.

Culture of sputum and of stomach washings.

Progress assessed by:—

X-ray.

Estimation of blood sedimentation rate.

Examination of sputum.

Assessment of weight and general condition.

Treatment

GENERAL

Isolation with full nursing care.

Improve nutrition to increase resistance.

A combination of rest and graduated exercises.

Plenty of fresh air.

Exposure to sunlight must be gradual.

When the fever has been absent for about 3 weeks, sitting out of bed for half an hour is allowed.

Diversional therapy in the form of craft work and later scholastic and social activities form an essential part of the long-term treatment.

SYMPTOMATIC

Oxygen, linctus, and sedatives.

For cough, a warm saline draught on waking to induce expectoration.

Bitter tonics or aperitifs are useful aids to appetite.

SPECIFIC

Streptomycin.

P.A.S. (Para-aminosalicylic acid).

Thiosemicarbazones.

Isoniazid.

SURGICAL

Collapse therapy by pneumothorax or a phrenic crush (the phrenic nerve supplying one side of the diaphragm is crushed at the base of the neck).

Lung resection.

INFLUENZA

An infectious disease with pyrexia.

Symptoms may involve either the breathing system or the gastro-intestinal tract.

It is caused by a virus.

Occurs in epidemics.

Has a short incubation period of a few days.

Symptoms are constitutional.

Sore throat with coryza (running eyes and nose) and a cough.

There are muscular pains in back and legs.

Temperature rises to about 104° F. (40° C.).

Treatment

GENERAL

Complete rest in bed until the temperature has been normal for 3 days and the patient is free of complications.

Light diet with fluids.

SYMPTOMATIC

Compound codeine tablets B.P. or paracetamol to relieve malaise and headache.

Decongestants, e.g., phenylephrine.

Caffeine to counteract low spirits.

SPECIFIC

None, although antibiotics may be given to prevent secondary infection, like pneumonia in the elderly.

Post-influenzal depression is quite a common occurrence.

CONGESTIVE HEART FAILURE

The heart fails to maintain an efficient circulation of blood.

Usually associated with old age.

The blood stagnates in the blood-vessels.

Organs throughout the body become congested with blood and tissue fluid, and every system in one way or another becomes involved.

Breathing is difficult and there is cyanosis.

Hypostatic pneumonia may result from lung congestion.

The pulse is weak, rapid, and often irregular.

Patient may feel sick and may vomit.

There is insomnia, restlessness, and sometimes confusion, and this seems to be worse at night.

Urinary output is diminished.

Oedema occurs throughout the body. In the early stages this may only affect the ankles, but gradually, fluid may collect in the cavities within the body and give rise to anasarca—generalized oedema.

There may be constipation or diarrhoea.

Agitation, restlessness, and apprehension are quite common, and even violent excitement is not unknown.

Treatment

GENERAL

Intensive nursing care in severe cases.

When the condition is of moderate severity, bed-rest with light diet. The patient is also propped up into a sitting position.

SYMPTOMATIC

Fluid intake is restricted.

Diuretics are important, e.g., saluric and aquamox.

Sodium restriction in the diet to reduce oedema.

Oxygen inhalations may be necessary.

Aminophylline may be given by slow intravenous injection. This increases heart action and dilates the coronary arteries. It also relaxes spasms of the bronchi. (Aminophylline may also be given as a suppository.)

SPECIFIC

None, although correction of cardiac irregularities if present with digoxin or by propranolol may be specific in a way.

CORONARY OCCLUSION

The coronary artery of the heart is blocked by a blood-clot.

This is an emergency. The patient may suddenly collapse and die.

There is a severe vice-like pain in the chest and upper abdomen which can last for days. Pain may come on at any time.

The patient becomes cyanosed and may vomit. He is anxious and restless.

Signs of shock appear and the blood-pressure falls.

Treatment

GENERAL

Absolute rest. Patient is not to strain at anything.

The patient should be put to bed with a minimum of effort.

If the heart stops, perform external cardiac massage and artificial respiration.

SYMPTOMATIC

Relief of pain is urgent.

A subcutaneous injection of morphine is given for this purpose.

Oxygen inhalations in 90–100 per cent concentration are used routinely.

Vasodilators may be administered.

Defibrillation with the use of artificial pace-maker may become necessary.

Pulmonary oedema is treated by digitalis, diuretics, and oxygen.

SPECIFIC
None.
The four main drugs of cardiac resuscitation are:—
Adrenaline.
Isoprenaline.
Calcium chloride.
Sodium bicarbonate.

ANAEMIA

This is a blood disorder due to insufficient number of normal red blood-cells. There are four main varieties:—

Deficiency anaemia due to lack of iron, vitamin B_{12} (as in pernicious anaemia), or other substances essential for the normal formation of red blood-cells.

Haemolytic anaemia due to the destruction of red blood-cells.

Aplastic anaemia arising from the failure of red blood-cell formation in the bone-marrow.

Agranulocytic anaemia due to a reduction in both red and white blood-cells. (Look up the meaning of *agranulocytosis* in your dictionary.)

General Signs and Symptoms Common to Most Anaemias

Pallor.
Weakness and tiredness.
Shortness of breath.
Loss of appetite, nausea, and vomiting.
Loss of interest.
Slight oedema of ankles.
Disturbed sleep.
Constipation.

Other Symptoms Peculiar to Specific Types of Anaemias include:—

Spooning of the nails and a smooth tongue in iron deficiency anaemia.

Soreness of the tongue with a yellowish skin, tingling sensations and numbness in legs, and achlorhydria in pernicious anaemia.

Haemorrhage into skin and from mucous membrane in aplastic anaemia.

Ulceration in mouth and throat in agranulocytic anaemia.

Treatment

GENERAL

Bed-rest in the early stages with full nursing care.
Attention to general health.

SYMPTOMATIC

Fresh air and sunlight and a good diet are all essential.
Aperitifs.
Mild hypnotics to aid a restful sleep.
Local treatment to sore mouth and throat.

SPECIFIC

Remove the cause.
Correct any deficiency: iron in iron deficiency anaemia, vitamin B_{12} in pernicious anaemia.
Blood transfusions.

LEUKAEMIA

A blood disorder due to the failure of the bone-marrow to produce sufficient number of normal white blood-cells, red cells, and platelets. A large number of abnormal white blood-cells are produced instead, and these accumulate in the blood.

The body's resistance to infection is lowered.

The person is therefore susceptible to many forms of infection.

Anaemia occurs due to lack of red blood-cells.

Haemorrhage may occur due to lack of platelets.

Acute leukaemia is a fatal disease lasting only a few weeks, whilst *chronic* leukaemia may last a number of years.

The spleen and the lymphatic glands are enlarged in both forms.

Gums and throat may ulcerate.

Treatment

GENERAL

Reassurance and good nursing.

SYMPTOMATIC

Blood transfusions.
Drugs:—
    Antipurines, e.g., mercaptopurine.
    Antifolic acid, e.g., methotrexate.
    Corticosteroids to reduce the number of white blood-cells.
    Antibiotics for infections.
    Hypnotics for insomnia.
    Analgesics for the relief of pain.

SPECIAL
None.

PEPTIC ULCERATION

There are three main types:—
Gastric in the stomach.
Duodenal in the duodenum.
Anastomostic at a juncture between two parts of the gut joined at an operation.
Contrast between the symptoms of gastric and duodenal ulcers:—

Gastric	*Duodenal*
Pain on taking food.	Pain when the stomach is empty.
Pain may be referred to the shoulder.	Pain is referred to the back between the shoulder blades.
There is loss of body-weight.	Pain is relieved by taking a small quantity of food such as milk and biscuits at frequent intervals.
Heartburn is common.	No apparent loss of weight.
	No heart burn.

There is tenderness in the epigastrium in both.
Haematemesis and melaena with anaemia may complicate both conditions.
Patients who suffer from peptic ulceration seem miserable and dejected and are quite likely to become depressed.

Treatment

GENERAL
Attention to health overall.
Systemic and prolonged medical treatment should be tried in every case of peptic ulcer.
Enlist the co-operation of the patient.
Patient remains in bed for a few weeks.
Smoking and alcohol are forbidden.
Should be free from business worry, and so on.
Rest and relaxation are vital.
Diet to be bland, high calorie, and given in small quantities at frequent intervals.
SYMPTOMATIC
Relieve pain by the use of antispasmodics, e.g., probanthine and biogastrone.

Antacids such as aluminium hydroxide 4- to 6-hourly are usually administered.

Intragastric milk-feeds with vitamin C may aid healing.

SPECIFIC

None, other than surgery in selected cases.

ACUTE APPENDICITIS

Invariably comes on suddenly, and if pain is severe, there is bound to be shock.

There is nausea and vomiting with a variable degree of constitutional disturbance, e.g., fever and increased pulse-rate.

Pain is present, and whilst this may start off as a generalized abdominal colic, it later becomes localized in the right iliac fossa.

Treatment

GENERAL

Bed-rest and combat shock.

SYMPTOMATIC

Relieve pain if severe, but use morphine wisely.

Pethedine may be the drug of choice.

SPECIFIC

Appendicectomy.

INTESTINAL OBSTRUCTION

Causes

Strangulated hernia.

Twisting of the gut by adhesions.

Carcinoma.

Chronic constipation.

Paralysis of the gut as in paralytic ileus.

One piece of gut being pushed into itself like a telescope.

A matted bolus of undigested food.

Signs and Symptoms

Pain.

Copious vomiting, the vomit being either green, yellow, or brown.

Abdominal distension.

Signs of dehydration are common, and these include a dry tongue, inelastic skin, sometimes thirst, and a general feeling of weakness.

Treatment

GENERAL

Bed-rest with full nursing care.

SYMPTOMATIC

Prepare to give an intravenous drip, and to pass a gastric aspirating tube. Aspirating the stomach prevents vomiting in this particular instance. If vomiting occurred there would always be a danger that the patient might inhale some of it into his lungs.

SPECIFIC

Surgery to remove the obstruction or to by-pass it as with a colostomy.

Abdominal disease is conducive to depression, hypochondria, and gloomy introspection.

DYSENTERY

Inflammation of the colon with ulceration, and caused in this country by a variety of bacilli, e.g., Sonne (mild), Flexner (intermediate in severity), Shiga (severe).

It has an incubation period of up to a week and is an epidemic disease.

Its incidence is directly related to the fly season.

Signs and Symptoms

Griping pains followed by diarrhoea.

The stools are foul and contain blood and mucus.

Constitutional symptoms are also present.

Treatment

GENERAL

Bed-rest with full nursing care.

Isolation.

Send a specimen of stools or a rectal swab for bacteriological diagnosis.

Give plenty of fluids.

SYMPTOMATIC

Apply warmth to the abdomen to relieve pain.

SPECIFIC

Sulphonamides.

Tetracyclines.

COLIC

A severe griping pain which comes in spasms, and is due to a sudden distension of a muscular tube such as the small intestine, ureter, and common bile-duct.

The pain is generalized in intestinal colic, shoots down to the thigh in renal colic, and shoots up to the shoulder-blades in biliary colic. With each bout of pain the person doubles up in agony and is shocked. In biliary colic, however, the pain tends to build up in intensity rather than come in waves.

Treatment

GENERAL

Bed-rest.

Give plenty of fluids.

In renal colic report if a stone is passed, and send a midstream specimen of urine to the laboratory.

SYMPTOMATIC

Relieve pain by giving pethedine (100 mg.) or morphine (15–30 mg.).

Atropine, an antispasmodic, may be used in order to counteract the spasm caused by pethedine and morphine.

Local heat may be applied to the area where pain is felt.

SPECIFIC

Remove the cause.

JAUNDICE

This is a condition in which there is an excess of bilirubin in the blood and tissues of the body. There are three main forms:—

Haemolytic, due to the destruction of red blood-cells.

Obstructive, due to blocking of the common bile-duct.

Toxic, due to liver damage by drugs.

Signs and Symptoms

Yellow pigmentation of the skin and mucous membrane. of The skin also itches.

In obstructive jaundice the stools are pale, due to the absence bile.

Urine, however, is dark in all forms.

Constitutional symptoms may be present if there is infection.

The pulse is slow (quite an exception to that expected with an infection).

There is nausea and vomiting.

The patient tends to be low spirited, even to the point of being depressed.

Treatment

GENERAL

Isolation if the cause is infective.

Complete bed-rest with full nursing care, and plenty of fluids.

SYMPTOMATIC

Fat-free diet.

Alkalis and bitters to allay nausea and to promote appetite.

Antihistamine may be used to overcome the itchiness. Calamine may also help.

SPECIFIC

Remove the cause.

Blood transfusions in haemolytic jaundice.

Corticosteroids if the condition is due to hepatitis.

Surgery in selected cases.

ACUTE NEPHRITIS

Acute inflammation of the kidneys.

Constitutional symptoms are present and there is also oedema of face, ankles, and lumbar regions.

Pain in the loins.

Urine output is diminished, and it may contain blood and albumen.

Treatment

GENERAL

Complete bed-rest and nursing care for about 6 weeks.

Restrict fluid intake in the early stages, but increase gradually as the urine output improves.

Salt is omitted.

Low protein diet at first.

Keep the urine alkaline with fruit juices, citrates, and bi-carbonates.

Ensure a daily bowel action.

Send a midstream specimen to the laboratory.

SYMPTOMATIC

Mild hypnotics if sleep is difficult.

Warmth to the loins.

SPECIFIC
  Drugs:—
    Penbritin (a variety of penicillin).
    Nitrofurantoin.

PYELITIS

Inflammation of the pelvis of the kidney.
Constitutional symptoms are present.
Pain in the loins.
Scalding and frequent micturition.
Acid urine.

Treatment

GENERAL
  Bed-rest with full nursing care.
  Plenty of fluids.
  Send a midstream specimen of urine to the laboratory.
SYMPTOMATIC
  Render urine alkaline by giving potassium citrate.
  Apply warmth to the loins.
SPECIFIC
  Drugs:—
    Sulphonamides.
    Penicillin.
    Negram.
    Tetracyclines.

CYSTITIS

Inflammation of the urinary bladder.
May occur at any age.
More common in women than men.
There is frequent micturition with a scalding sensation.
Pain in the lower abdomen.
Constitutional symptoms common.

Treatment

GENERAL
  Send a midstream specimen of urine to the laboratory.
  Bed-rest with full nursing care and plenty of fluids.
SYMPTOMATIC
  Keep urine alkaline.
  Warmth to lower abdomen.

SPECIFIC

Sulphonamides.

Penicillin for staphylococcal infection.

Colistin for pyocyaneus infection.

Cycloserine for coliform organisms.

DIABETES MELLITUS

A metabolic disturbance due to lack of insulin. This results in hyperglycaemia (excess sugar in the blood), in incomplete combustion of fat, and in ketosis—the presence in the blood of acid substances called ketones, which are derived from fat. Fat cannot be completely metabolized because there is no sugar available for its oxidation. Sugar is in turn lacking because there is no insulin secreted to contain it in the liver.

Signs and Symptoms

Polyuria: increased output of urine.

Glycosuria: sugar in the urine.

Ketonuria: ketones in the urine.

Ketones are also excreted in the breath—that is why it has a sweet smell.

There is thirst to make good the water lost in the urine and to flush the excess sugar and ketones from the blood.

The mouth is dry and the tongue becomes 'beefy' in appearance.

Itchiness of the genitals is common.

There is loss of weight and a general feeling of weakness.

There may be a rapid pulse with epigastric pain.

If untreated the patient becomes more and more drowsy and finally becomes comatose.

Diabetes may be accompanied by irritability, agitation, and depression, especially when there is a marked degree of acidosis.

Treatment

GENERAL

Rest in bed with routine nursing care if the condition is severe. Maintain a high standard of personal cleanliness.

SYMPTOMATIC

Cleanliness of genitalia.

Care of the mouth.

Plenty of drinking water to be available.

SPECIFIC

Stabilization:—

Estimation of blood-sugar level.

Routine testing of urine for glucose and ketones.

Dieting—low calorie to start with.

Lawrence Line Ration Diet is an alternative.

Insulin required for most patients.

Tablets such as tolbutamide may control mild diabetes.

REHABILITATION

Reassurance.

Educate to accept the condition.

Train to give injections and to weigh food and so on.

Train to accept limitation of activities which the disorder imposes.

Not to look upon himself as an invalid.

Hyperglycaemia

Associated with a diabetic patient who is having too much sugar or not enough insulin.

Breath smells sweet, like nail-varnish remover.

Cheeks are often flushed.

Pulse not unduly fast, but strong.

Urine contains a lot of sugar.

Loss of consciousness.

This condition develops gradually. (See also symptoms of diabetes mellitus.)

Hypoglycaemia

Associated with a diabetic patient who is having too much insulin.

Breath does not smell sweet.

Cheeks and skin in general are pale, moist, and cold.

Pulse increased in rate and weak.

Urine contains no sugar.

Loss of consciousness.

This condition comes on quickly. Usually the patient is seen to act strangely. Some may become silly and over-talkative while others may become morose and truculent. The treatment is to give sugar by mouth as soon as possible. Without sugar the patient may, before losing consciousness, become confused, noisy, and extremely excited.

Always seek medical aid

ACIDOSIS	ALKALOSIS
A condition in which there is excess acid in the blood, as in diabetes mellitus if untreated. It may also be associated with taking too many aspirins.	A condition in which the blood is more alkaline than normal. Associated with over-breathing in hysteria. Taking too much alkali by mouth as in the treatment of stomach upsets. Prolonged vomiting.
The main symptoms are a fast pulse, cold sweating extremities, over-breathing, hyper-noea, and vomiting.	Some of the earliest symptoms are lassitude, drowsiness, irritability, loss of appetite, and nausea.

The essential in both conditions is to treat the underlying cause.

PERIPHERAL NEURITIS

May be found in alcoholism, in various toxic states, and as a complication of diabetes mellitus.

There is pain, tingling, and numbness in limbs.

Diminished or altered sensations.

Muscular wasting resulting in foot drop and wrist drop.

Treatment

GENERAL
  Rest.

SYMPTOMATIC
  Analgesics.
  Prevent deformity by splinting.

SPECIFIC
  Remove the cause.
  Vitamin B.
  Electrical treatment.
  Passive and later active exercises.

Peripheral neuritis is quite a common symptom in the mental condition known as *Korsakow's syndrome*. This is a condition in which there are illusions and hallucinations. Memory is also poor and, in an attempt to fill the memory gaps, the patient gives the most circumstantial account of events, which are entirely the figment of his imagination.

CEREBROVASCULAR ACCIDENTS

Cerebral Haemorrhage	Thrombosis	Embolism
Sudden onset and more common in the elderly than the young. Popularly referred to as a stroke.	Gradual onset, preceded by a headache, progressive over hours.	Sudden onset at any age. No warning signs.

Symptoms are variable according to the severity and the area of the brain affected.

There may be aphasia (loss of speech) or dysphasia (difficult speech).

Visual or sensory loss.

Convulsions.

Fever.

Stiff neck.

Paralysis of varying degrees, e.g., hemiparesis (partial paralysis of one side of the body), hemiplegia (complete paralysis of one side of the body).

If in coma, the patient may die or recover partially or completely.

Mental impairment and emotional instability often persist.

Treatment

GENERAL

Graded nursing care, ranging from intensive care to convalescence.

SYMPTOMATIC

Occasional splinting to prevent deformity.

If speech is lost, use tact in interpreting patient's wants.

SPECIFIC

Anticoagulants if diagnosis of thrombo-embolism is made.

Rehabilitation.

DISSEMINATED OR MULTIPLE SCLEROSIS

A chronic relapsing disease in which there is scattered degeneration of the motor tract.

There is tremor on movement—intentional tremor—with weakness, stiffness or jerking of legs, and ataxia.

There is blurred and double vision.

The speech is slurred and sometimes jerky.

There is emotional lability in the sense that the patient is emotionally unstable and easily upset.

As this is a progressive condition, the patient becomes an invalid and later bedridden.

Bed-sores, incontinence, urinary infection, and pneumonia may complicate the condition.

The average duration of life is about 20 years from onset.

Treatment

GENERAL

Reassurance, encouragement, tolerance, and patience.

Attention to general hygiene.

Progressive nursing care.

SYMPTOMATIC

Physiotherapy.

Orthopaedic appliances to aid movement.

Prevent fatigue, but keep the patient active as long as possible.

SPECIFIC

None.

HIGHLIGHTS OF SOME NOTABLE DIFFERENCES BETWEEN:—

Hypertension	Hypotension
Associated with:—	Associated with:—
Arteriosclerosis (hardening of the arteries with advancing age).	Addison's disease. Vasomotor instability. Shock.
Kidney disease.	Heart failure.
Increased intracranial pressure.	Anaemia.
Polycythaemia (increase in the number of red blood-cells).	Drugs.
Headaches, giddiness, ringing in the ears are common symptoms.	General weakness, giddiness and faintness, numbness and pallor of extremities are common symptoms.
Moodiness with amnesia and confusion, however, may complicate the picture.	Depression and irritability may also occur.

Essential to correct the underlying causes in both conditions.

Hypertension can be controlled by the use of a number of specific drugs, such as Aldomet, Inversine, Reserpine.

Apart from vasoconstrictors, only drugs which serve to correct the underlying cause are of use in hypertension.

Asthma (paroxysmal dyspnoea with short inspiration and long wheezing expiration)

BRONCHIAL

A sizeable percentage shows evidence of hypersensitivity to ingestion of certain foods or to inhalation of pollens, feathers, moulds, dust, etc.

May occur at any time of the day or night. Has a sudden onset. Emotion may precipitate an attack. An attack may be treated either by an inhalation of adrenaline 1 in 100 or by the use of an isoprenaline spray. Resistant cases respond to either aminophylline or hydrocortisone intravenously. Morphine is to be avoided.

CARDIAC (referred to today as acute pulmonary oedema)

Due to a failing left ventricle. Attacks usually at night. Made worse by use of hypnotics. There is a sudden onset of dyspnoea. The patient sits up in bed or walks to the window. Morphine is more satisfactory than barbiturates in its control.

Oxygen inhalations and an intravenous injection of aminophylline cut short an attack.

RENAL

Associated with uraemia and when there is acidosis and circulatory failure. Dyspnoea may be paroxysmal or continuous. Correcting the acidosis with the administration of oxygen and morphine gives some relief.

Hyperthyroidism

An endocrine disturbance due to over-secretion of the hormone thyroxine. The excess thyroxine circulating in the blood increases metabolism.

Hypothyroidism

An endocrine disturbance due to under-secretion of thyroxine. The complete absence of thyroxine produces *myxoedema*.

The body is over-stimulated in general and loses weight. Pulse-rate is increased. Palpitations are present. The body is hot and there is a good deal of sweating. The patient feels nervy and jittery and has a fine involuntary tremor of all muscles. The eyes protrude and stare.

The specific treatment for this involves either the administration of radioactive iodine or the surgical removal of some of the gland.

Symptoms of hypothyroidism in general are the opposite to those found under hyperthyroidism. Metabolic activity slows down. Body-weight increases. The pulse is slow. Mentally the patient is slow and dull. Eyes are puffy. The nose tends to be red whilst the rest of the face is pale. Body temperature is low and the skin is always dry.

Thyroid extract by mouth corrects this condition.

Skin Complaints

SCABIES

This is due to the presence of a spider-like group of parasites called *ascarus*. The female burrows under the skin to lay her eggs.

The common areas of skin affected are those between the fingers and around the wrists. As the female burrows she sets up irritation and this causes scratching.

The patient, after having been thoroughly bathed, is painted all over with benzyl benzoate emulsion. Clothing and bedding are disinfected.

RINGWORM

A contagious skin condition caused by a fungus.

It appears as a red dry itching spot which if left untreated enlarges progressively. Any part of the body may be affected.

A few applications of either iodine, Whitfield ointment, Tineafax ointment, or Tinaderm cream is the treatment of choice. Resistant cases may be treated by the administration of Griseofulvin, an antifungal drug, either orally or by injection.

IMPETIGO

This is a contagious complaint. Common in young children. Caused by a streptococcus. The crusts which form may contain staphyloccoci.

PSORIASIS

Not a contagious condition. Common in middle and old age. Cause unknown.

Starts with the appearance of small red spots. As these

Small blisters containing pus appear. These burst and crusts form. The surrounding skin is inflamed.

Advisable to remove the crusts before applying a suitable antibiotic, e.g., neomycin. Patients will need their own face flannels and towels. With adequate treatment it clears up quickly.

enlarge they join up with each other and become covered with silvery-looking scales. It is a dry eruption. The commonest sites affected are the elbows and knees.

Application of ointment containing either chrysarobin or coal tar is the standard treatment, still in use. Corticosteroids are sometimes tried. An extremely difficult complaint to get rid of.

CLINICAL ASPECTS OF NURSING THE SICK

1. Attend to the bed. Have a soft mattress. Make sure that the rubber if any is soft, smooth, and free from creases. Linen to be free from creases and darns, particularly those that come into direct contact with the patient's skin. Blankets placed next to the patient to be non-irritating. Use the softer kind. Bedclothes to be light and warm and not too tight. Use cradles if the patient is weak or helpless.

2. Patient's back to be well supported.

3. Pillows to be arranged so that there is a soft one next to the patient.

4. Pillows to be turned over from time to time to give a cool surface to lie on.

5. Helpless patients to be turned from side to side every 2 hours.

6. Routine attention to pressure areas every 4 hours.

7. Attention to oral hygiene before and/or after food or meals.

8. General cleanliness. Wash the patient's face at least twice a day and hair at least once a week. After grooming let the patient look in the mirror.

9. Be gentle when inserting bedpans.

10. Avoid exposing the patient too much.

11. Ensure that the environment is sweet smelling and generally comfortable. Consider ventilation, heating, and lighting.

12. See that the patient is in the most comfortable position and easy to attend to.

13. Anticipate his wants and try to attend to these immediately.

14. Make food and tray for serving attractive, and serve food daintily.

15. Reduce noise to a minimum.

16. Keep the patient from being lonely and allow time for a chat with him from time to time.

17. Avoid being too fussy, and guard against setting a standard which is too demanding and inhibiting.

18. Check to see that bandages, splints, etc. are not too tight.

19. Make sure that the equipment for the patient's personal use is at hand, e.g., a sputum mug.

20. Aim to give clear instructions and to inform the patient of your intentions and expectations.

21. Help him with such tasks as letter writing and general interests.

22. At all times adopt the best nursing technique in all that you do.

23. Be extra quiet at night. Shade glaring lights. Visit him frequently to see that all is well.

24. Comfort if he cannot sleep and offer reassurance.

25. At all times take things calmly and avoid flustering.

26. Always be on the look out for the small things that he may want, e.g., spectacles or dentures.

27. Show respect to visitors. Be courteous and try not to keep them waiting unnecessarily.

28. Give drugs and medicines to time.

29. Ensure that you yourself are clean, tidy, attractive, and pleasant.

30. Consider the patient's general position in the ward. This should be accessible, pleasant, and acceptable to the patient.

31. Respect his beliefs and faith, and always be kind and respectful.

FEATURES OF ROUTINE CLINICAL NURSING

General Treatment

Nursing care of a bedridden patient varies according to the degree and the severity of the illness. During the acute phase of a serious illness it would be intensive, with nursing care concentrated on the patient throughout the 24 hours. As the patient improves, however, care would become less concentrated and would therefore be graduated to the patient's immediate needs.

Nursing Care of a Bedridden Patient involves Consideration of:—

Bed: Bed-making at least twice a day.

Position in bed: Placing and maintaining the patient in the most comfortable and suitable position in bed.

Pressure areas: Care of pressure areas 4-hourly at least.

Movement: Moving the patient from side to side, every 2 hours if helpless.

Exercise: Encouraging deep-breathing exercises to minimize the risk of hypostatic pneumonia. Passive exercise of the limbs if the patient is unable to move these by himself.

Morale and comfort: Fostering morale, interest, and general comfort (see suggestions on how to make a bedridden patient comfortable on previous page).

Cleanliness: Washing, bathing, and grooming.

Nourishment: Feeding and supplying adequate nourishment.

Observation: Continuous observation of the patient's appearance, position, comfort, and so on.

Excreta: Checking urine output, bowel action, and sputum expectorated.

Anticipation of wants: Arranging that all facilities are available to satisfy the immediate physical wants of the patient.

Conscientiousness in keeping charts, records, and reports. Interpreting and carrying out instructions. Making sure that the patient receives the treatment and drugs prescribed to time.

Nursing techniques: Practising the correct techniques of lifting, feeding, of inserting a bed-pan, and so on.

Ill Effects of lying in Bed for a Long Time

  i. Muscle weakness.
 ii. Loss of body-weight.
iii. Pressure sores.
 iv. Stiffness of joints.
  v. Hypostatic pneumonia.
 vi. Cystitis (due to incomplete emptying of bladder).
vii. Constipation and flatulence.
viii. General discomfort.
 ix. Low morale and restlessness.
  x. Loss of appetite.
 xi. Insomnia and distress especially at night.

WARD REPORTING

Points to Emphasize

1. Reports should be brief and to the point. Reports, however, should contain:—

   a. Description of a situation or condition as it stands.

   b. Events since last report.

   c. Present events.

   d. Future requirements.

2. The nurse should not copy the doctor's records but should report on the observations of the nursing staff.

3. Writing must be legible and *abbreviations avoided*.

4. Spellings must be accurate as mistakes may give wrong information, especially about drugs which have similar names.

5. *All reports are signed by the person writing the report* and alterations initialled and reported to the nursing officer concerned.

6. Where a duplicate book is used, the duplicate copy has to be legible and any alterations initialled on both copies.

7. It is advisable to keep reports for at least 5 years.

8. A report should be given to all nursing staff as they report for duty. Before allowing the ward staff to read a written report, it is always wise for the nurse in charge to give an oral report first. In this way she can emphasize more fully what she considers are the important essentials.

9. Student nurses should always read the day and night reports to make themselves fully conversant with what goes on on the ward and they should always be present at 'handovers'.

10. It is the responsibility of each nurse to keep her colleagues informed of the various changes which have taken place on the ward.

Information regarding the condition of patients should preferably be given by the nurse in charge.

The nurse should avoid holding long conversations with patients' relatives, and questions from relatives are best left for the nurse in charge to answer.

ANSWERING THE TELEPHONE

It is surprising how casual and indifferent some people are about this.

Method

Lift receiver, give name of Ward/Department, and state name of person answering, e.g., 'Ward 12. Nurse Smith speaking'.

Any message should be taken down in writing and repeated to the person at the other end of the telephone. Also, avoid long conversations on the telephone, as someone might want the ward urgently.

DRUGS

Side-effects	Toxic Effects
Specific physiological disturbances without structural damage.	Great risk of irreparable structural damage.
Autonomic nervous system involved first. Physiological disturbance may follow.	Affect structures directly.
Inconvenient but not particularly dangerous, need to restrict dosage only in the average circumstances.	Dangerous. Not easily reversible. Need to stop the drug.
Precipitating factors few if any.	Precipitating factors enhancing toxic effect, e.g., degree of tolerance, metabolism, rate of excretion, and accumulative effect.
Examples of side-effects: dry mouth, hypotension, tremors.	Examples of toxic effect: skin rashes, jaundice, anaemia, Parkinsonism.

Pharmacy and Poisons Act, 1933, regulates the supply of poisons.

Dangerous drugs are regulated by the *Dangerous Drugs Act*, 1951 and 1967:—

SCHEDULE I (lists all the drugs):—

Drugs of addiction:—

Morphine	Pethedrine
Heroin	Physeptone
Cocaine	

Miscellaneous:—

Atropine	Dover's powder
Digoxin	Eserine
Barium	Picrotoxin
Ergotamine	Philocarpine
Hyoscine	Codeine tablets
Belladonna	

SCHEDULE IV (lists only a selection of drugs; a medical prescription is required to obtain Schedule IV drugs):—

Part A:—
Barbiturates (seconal, phenobarbitone, amytal).
Cytotoxics (mustine).
Digoxin.

Part B:—
Non-barbiturate hypnotics (glutethimide, propiomazine, methaqualone).
Oral hypoglycaemics (tolbutamide).
Antihistamines (diphenhydramine).
Sulphonamides (sulphadiazine).
Antidepressants (phenelzine).
Tranquillizers (chlorpromazine).
Pituitary extracts (vasopressin).
Miscellaneous (benzedrine, adrenaline).

Drugs not covered by the Pharmacy and Poisons Act, or covered on minor points with reference to labelling:—

Ephedrine	Coramine
Amyl nitrite	Aminophylline
Insulin	Anticoagulants

Novocaine (less than 10 per cent)

Therapeutic Substances Act, 1956, controls the sale and supply of:—
Antibiotics (penicillin, tetracyclines, streptomycin).
Cortisone.
Sera and vaccines.

The Administration of Medicines and Drugs by Mouth

The mouth is the most common route used. Medicines are generally looked upon as non-poisonous, and drugs as poisonous. A selected number of drugs are described as dangerous in that they are drugs of addiction. These include opium and its preparations, cocaine, morphine, heroin, Indian hemp, pethedine, Amidone and Physeptone (methadone), Heptalgin (phenadoxone).

Each dose administered must be entered in a special register, with the date, the name of the doctor who prescribed it, the patient's name, the name and dose of the drug, the time of giving the drug, the name of the nurse giving it, and the name of the person who checked it (one of the last two has to be a Registered nurse).

No medicine or drug should be given to a patient unless prescribed by a doctor. It is also the doctor's responsibility to write up medicine and treatment cards. This is not the nurse's job.

Rules for the Administration of Medicines and Drugs

1. The label on each container should be carefully read, and the nurse should follow the instructions given. If there is any doubt, she should not hesitate to consult the nurse in charge. This of course applies mainly to trainee nurses.

2. No medicine or drug should be given from a container which is not clearly labelled.

3. The label should be checked four times: before taking the container from the cupboard; just before taking the medicine or drug from its container—or pouring it out as the case may be; after it has been taken out of its container; and before giving it to the patient. Check to make sure that you have the right medicine, the right patient, the right dose, and the right time.

4. A bottle with sediment has to be shaken and the liquid stirred before giving.

5. Administer to time.

6. Never use a medicine or a drug which has been left out of its container.

7. Never return it to its container if it is not taken, and always record it if this occurs. (Unused drugs must always be returned to the dispensary, and from time to time, perhaps weekly, the medicine cards should be checked against the record of the drugs given and those not given.)

8. Try not to handle tablets, pills, and cachets with the hands. Use a teaspoon.

9. In a psychiatric hospital especially, never leave a medicine trolley unattended, or the medicine cupboard open without someone there.

10. Never administer a medicine or drug by mouth to a semi-conscious patient.

The Administration

Use a small tray for a patient who is unable to collect his medicine or drug, or when a medicine trolley is not used.

Carry out the instructions as listed.

Set out to make the procedure pleasant for the patient. The nurse's approach and attitude are all important. An awkward approach could make a patient reject what has been offered.

A number of patients may need a lot of persuasion. How does one persuade a patient to take his medicine if he does not want it ? (Refer to the Art of Suggestion on p. 49.)

Observe the reactions of the patient to taking the medicine or drug. Was he pleased ? Did he express any opinions ? Be ready to report your observations either to the doctor or to the nurse in charge.

With some patients, especially the weak and the old, or the stubborn, it may be advisable to pour a liquid medicine, once measured, into a feeding cup.

Always stay with the patient until you are quite certain that it has been taken.

Afterwards make sure that everything is cleared up and put back in its appropriate place. This makes for efficiency and lessens risks. One cannot be too careful where drugs are involved.

Care of the Medicine Cupboard

1. Orderly arrangement of bottles, etc.
2. To be inspected daily.
3. All drugs and medicine to be in their proper container, and correctly labelled.
4. No drug in powder form or tablet form to be left wrapped in paper.
5. Poisons to be kept separate from non-poisons.
6. External applications to be separate from internal medicaments.
7. Cupboards, containers, and labels to be kept clean.
8. Empty bottles, etc., to be removed.
9. Note expiry date for certain drugs.
10. Ensure that contents are covered—cork in situ, etc.
11. No unauthorized person to have access to the cupboard.
12. Keys to be kept with the person in charge of the ward.
13. Storing of stock bottles of medicine not often used to be discouraged.
14. Observe any special instruction regarding storage and inspection of drugs.
15. Note the separate compartments for D.D.A., Schedule I and Schedule IV poisons.

INDEX